Celiac Disease

Editors

BENJAMIN LEBWOHL
PETER H.R. GREEN

GASTROENTEROLOGY CLINICS OF NORTH AMERICA

www.gastro.theclinics.com

Consulting Editor
ALAN L. BUCHMAN

March 2019 • Volume 48 • Number 1

ELSEVIER

1600 John F. Kennedy Boulevard • Suite 1800 • Philadelphia, Pennsylvania, 19103-2899
http://www.theclinics.com

GASTROENTEROLOGY CLINICS OF NORTH AMERICA Volume 48, Number 1
March 2019 ISSN 0889-8553, ISBN-13: 978-0-323-65523-1

Editor: Kerry Holland
Developmental Editor: Sara Watkins

Gastroenterology Clinics of North America (ISSN 0889-8553) is published quarterly by Elsevier Inc., 360 Park Avenue South, New York, NY 10010-1710. Months of issue are March, June, September, and December. Business and Editorial Offices: 1600 John F. Kennedy Blvd., Suite 1800, Philadelphia, PA 19103-2899. Customer Service Office: 6277 Sea Harbor Drive, Orlando, FL 32887-4800. Periodicals postage paid at New York, NY and additional mailing offices. Subscription prices are $361.00 per year (US individuals), $100.00 per year (US students), $692.00 per year (US institutions), $387.00 per year (Canadian individuals), $220.00 per year (Canadian students), $849.00 per year (Canadian institutions), $463.00 per year (international individuals), $220.00 per year (international students), and $849.00 per year (international institutions). Foreign air speed delivery is included in all *Clinics* subscription prices. All prices are subject to change without notice. **POSTMASTER:** Send address changes to *Gastroenterology Clinics of North America*, Elsevier Health Sciences Division, Subscription Customer Service, 3251 Riverport Lane, Maryland Heights, MO 63043. **Telephone: 1-800-654-2452 (U.S. and Canada); 314-447-8871 (outside U.S. and Canada). Fax: 314-447-8029. E-mail: journalscustomerservice-usa@elsevier.com (for print support); journalsonlinesupport-usa@elsevier.com (for online support).**

Reprints. For copies of 100 or more, of articles in this publication, please contact the Commercial Reprints Department, Elsevier Inc., 360 Part Avenue South, New York, New York 10010-1710. Tel. 212-633-3874, Fax: 212-633-3820, E-mail: reprints@elsevier.com.

Gastroenterology Clinics of North America is also published in Italian by Il Pensiero Scientifico Editore, Rome, Italy; and in Portuguese by Interlivros Edicoes Ltda., Rua Commandante Coelho 1085, 21250 Cordovil, Rio de Janeiro, Brazil.

Gastroenterology Clinics of North America is covered in *MEDLINE/PubMed (Index Medicus), Excerpta Medica, Current Contents/Clinical Medicine, Science Citation Index, ISI/BIOMED*, and *BIOSIS*.

Contributors

CONSULTING EDITOR

ALAN L. BUCHMAN, MD, MSPH, FACN, FACG, FACP, AGAF
Medical Director, Health Care Services Corporation, Professor of Clinical Surgery and Medical Director, Intestinal Rehabilitation and Transplant Center, University of Illinois at Chicago, Chicago, Illinois, USA

EDITORS

BENJAMIN LEBWOHL, MD, MS
Assistant Professor of Medicine and Epidemiology, Director of Clinical Research, Celiac Disease Center at Columbia University Medical Center, New York, New York, USA

PETER H.R. GREEN, MD
Phyllis and Ivan Seidenberg Professor of Medicine, Director, Celiac Disease Center at Columbia University Medical Center, New York, New York, USA

AUTHORS

ARMIN ALAEDINI, PhD
Department of Medicine, Institute of Human Nutrition, Celiac Disease Center at Columbia University Medical Center, New York, New York, USA

JULIO C. BAI, MD
Professor Emeritus Research Institutes, School of Medicine, Consultant, "Dr. C. Bonorino Udaondo" Universidad del Salvador, Gastroenterology Hospital, ABB, CABA, Argentina

GOVIND BHAGAT, MD
Professor of Pathology and Cell Biology, Columbia University Irving Medical Center, NewYork-Presbyterian Hospital, New York, New York, USA

GIACOMO CAIO, MD
Department of Medical and Surgical Sciences, St. Orsola-Malpighi Hospital, University of Bologna, Bologna, Italy; Mucosal Immunology and Biology Research Center, Massachusetts General Hospital, Harvard Medical School, Boston, Massachusetts, USA

CARLO CATASSI, MD
Department of Pediatrics, Head, Center for Celiac Research, Università Politecnica delle Marche, Ancona, Ancona, Italy; Visiting Professor, Massachusetts General Hospital, Boston, Massachusetts, USA

CHRISTOPHE CELLIER, MD, PhD
Université Paris Descartes, Gastroenterology Department, Hôpital Européen Georges Pompidou, APHP, Inserm UMR1163, Paris, France

ROBERTO DE GIORGIO, MD
Department of Medical Sciences, Nuovo Arcispedale St. Anna in Cona, University of Ferrara, Ferrara, Italy

MELINDA DENNIS, MS, RDN, LD
Nutrition Coordinator, Celiac Center, Beth Israel Deaconess Medical Center, Boston, Massachusetts, USA

ALESSIO FASANO, MD
W. Allan Walker Chair of Pediatric Gastroenterology and Nutrition, Professor of Pediatrics, Harvard Medical School Chief of the Division of Pediatric Gastroenterology and Nutrition, Associate Chief, Department of Pediatrics, Basic, Clinical and Translational Research, Massachusetts General Hospital for Children, Celiac Research Program, Harvard Medical School, Boston, Massachusetts, USA

ISABEL A. HUJOEL, MD
Instructor in Medicine, Division of Gastroenterology and Hepatology, Mayo Clinic, Rochester, Minnesota, USA

STEFFEN HUSBY, MD, PhD
Professor, Hans Christian Andersen Children's Hospital, Odense University Hospital, Odense C, Denmark

CIARAN P. KELLY, MD
Professor, Department of Medicine, Beth Israel Deaconess Medical Center, Celiac Research Program, Harvard Medical School, Boston, Massachusetts, USA

SUNEETA KRISHNAREDDY, MD, MS
Assistant Professor of Medicine, Digestive and Liver Diseases, Columbia University, New York, New York, USA

STEPHEN M. LAGANA, MD
Assistant Professor of Pathology and Cell Biology, Columbia University Irving Medical Center, NewYork-Presbyterian Hospital, New York, New York, USA

ANNE R. LEE, EdD, RDN, LD
Instructor, Nutritional Medicine, Celiac Disease Center at Columbia University Medical Center, New York, New York, USA

DANIEL LEFFLER, MD, MS
Harvard Celiac Disease Research Program, Associate Professor, Department of Medicine, Division of Gastroenterology, Beth Israel Deaconess Medical Center, Takeda Pharmaceuticals, Boston, Massachusetts, USA

SUZANNE K. LEWIS, MD
Associate Professor of Medicine, Division of Digestive Diseases, Celiac Disease Center at Columbia University Medical Center, Columbia University, New York, New York, USA

JONAS F. LUDVIGSSON, MD, PhD
Department of Medical Epidemiology and Biostatistics, Karolinska Institutet, Solna, Sweden; Department of Pediatrics, Örebro University Hospital, Örebro, Sweden; Division of Epidemiology and Public Health, School of Medicine, University of Nottingham, City Hospital, Nottingham, United Kingdom; Department of Medicine, Celiac Disease Center at Columbia University Medical Center, Columbia University College of Physicians and Surgeons, New York, New York, USA

GOVIND K. MAKHARIA, MD, DM, DNB
Professor, Department of Gastroenterology and Human Nutrition, All India Institute of Medical Sciences, New Delhi, India

GEORGIA MALAMUT, MD, PhD
Université Paris Descartes, Gastroenterology Department, Hôpital Européen Georges Pompidou, APHP, Inserm UMR1163, Paris, France

ROBERTO MANFREDINI, MD
Department of Medical Sciences, Nuovo Arcispedale St. Anna in Cona, University of Ferrara, Ferrara, Italy

TARA McCARTHY, MS, RDN
Clinical Nutrition Specialist, Division of Gastroenterology, Hepatology and Nutrition, Celiac Center, Boston Children's Hospital, Boston, Massachusetts, USA

JOSEPH A. MURRAY, MD, PhD
Division of Gastroenterology and Hepatology, Department of Immunology, Mayo Clinic, Rochester, Minnesota, USA; University of Southern Denmark, Odense, Denmark

NORELLE R. REILLY, MD
Assistant Professor of Pediatrics, Division of Pediatric Gastroenterology, Columbia University Medicine Center, New York, New York, USA

ALBERTO RUBIO-TAPIA, MD
Assistant Professor of Medicine, Division of Gastroenterology and Hepatology, Mayo Clinic, Rochester, Minnesota, USA

CAROL E. SEMRAD, MD
Professor of Medicine, The University of Chicago, Chicago, Illinois, USA

GLORIA SERENA, PhD
Post-Doctoral Fellow, Massachusetts General Hospital for Children, Division of Pediatric Gastroenterology and Nutrition, Mucosal Immunology and Biology Research Center, Celiac Research Program, Harvard Medical School, Boston, Massachusetts, USA

JOCELYN A. SILVESTER, MD, PhD
Instructor of Pediatrics, Harvard Celiac Disease Research Program, Division of Gastroenterology and Nutrition, Boston Children's Hospital, Beth Israel Deaconess Medical Center, Boston, Massachusetts, USA; Max Rady College of Medicine, University of Manitoba, Winnipeg, Manitoba, Canada

PRASHANT SINGH, MB BS
Harvard Celiac Disease Research Program, Department of Medicine, Division of Gastroenterology, Beth Israel Deaconess Medical Center, Boston, Massachusetts, USA

MELANIE UHDE, PhD
Department of Medicine, Celiac Disease Center at Columbia University Medical Center, New York, New York, USA

UMBERTO VOLTA, MD
Department of Medical and Surgical Sciences, St. Orsola-Malpighi Hospital, University of Bologna, Bologna, Italy

Contents

> Celiac disease is a common, chronic inflammatory disorder of the small intestine triggered by exposure to gluten in individuals with certain genetic types. This disorder affects people of any age or gender. Although often thought to be European in origin, it is now global in extent. Presentations are variable, from asymptomatic patients to severe malnutrition. Initial detection usually relies on celiac-specific serology, and confirmation often requires intestinal biopsy. There have been substantial increases in prevalence and incidence over the last 2 decades for reasons that are almost certainly environmental but for which there is no clarity as to cause.

> The presentation in celiac disease is shifting from the classical malabsorptive presentation to more nonclassical presentations, requiring clinicians to maintain a high level of suspicion for the disease and to be aware of the possible extraintestinal manifestations. The diagnosis of celiac disease is guided by initial screening with serology, followed by confirmation with an upper endoscopy and small intestinal biopsy. In some pediatric cases, biopsy may be avoided.

> Celiac disease is a common immune-mediated disorder that occurs in individuals with permissive genetics (HLA-DQ2/DQ8 genotype) following exposure to certain wheat proteins. The histopathologic manifestations of small intestinal mucosal injury (villus atrophy, crypt hyperplasia, and intraepithelial lymphocytosis) are well recognized. However, these findings are not specific for celiac disease, because they are observed in other small intestinal disorders. These mimics include common and rare entities, the list of which continues to grow. This article discusses the histopathology and differential diagnosis of celiac disease and provides the pathologist's perspective on biopsy adequacy, evaluation, and reporting in light of current knowledge.

Celiac disease (CD) is an autoimmune-related disease causing inflammation in the small intestine triggered by the ingestion of gluten in the diet. The gluten-free diet (GFD) is the only treatment. Nutritional deficiencies of macronutrients and micronutrients are frequently found in untreated or newly diagnosed CD. A registered dietitian nutritionist is uniquely qualified to educate on the GFD and assess and support nutritional status at diagnosis and long term as well as helping patients with nonresponsive CD. Quality of life is important to address in individuals with CD because the GFD affects all aspects of life.

Celiac disease predominantly involves the proximal small bowel, but villus atrophy can be patchy, spare the duodenum, and be present more distally. Video capsule endoscopy is more sensitive than standard endoscopy to detect villus atrophy, and can define extent of disease, though it cannot obtain biopsies. Duodenal biopsy is the gold standard for diagnosis. Video capsule endoscopy assists in special circumstances when biopsy is not possible, and in equivocal diagnosis. Video capsule endoscopy and enteroscopy are recommended for evaluating complicated celiac disease, especially refractory celiac disease type II. Future developments include computer-assisted capsule programs and advanced capsule and enteroscope design.

There is an unmet need for diagnostic and treatment interventions for celiac disease. Both clinical trials and real-world studies require careful selection of clinical outcome measures. Often, neither serology nor histology is an appropriate primary outcome. This article reviews various measures of intestinal function and nutrition, patient-reported outcome measures for symptoms and for health-related quality of life, and measures of sickness burden as they apply to intervention studies for celiac disease. A series of case studies is presented to illustrate key considerations in selecting outcome measures for dietary interventions, pharmacologic interventions, and real-world studies.

Celiac disease, once thought to be very uncommon in Asia, is now emerging in many Asian countries. Although the absolute number of patients with celiac disease at present is not very high, this number is expected to increase markedly over the next few years/decades owing to increasing awareness. It is now that the medical community across the Asia should define the extent of the problem and prepare to handle the impending epidemic of celiac disease in Asia.

The healthy microbiome is necessary for normal immune development in the gut. Alterations in the microbial makeup after a critical window increase the risk of autoimmunity, including celiac disease. Although this dysbiosis has been described in adult and pediatric patients, factors leading to dysbiosis are still being elucidated. Genetics has some role in determining the microbiome makeup of the host, but other factors have yet to be determined. The microbiome remains an important therapeutic target in many autoimmune conditions, including celiac disease, however studies have yet to determine the ideal replacement therapy to correct the dysbiosis.

Currently, the only effective treatment for celiac disease is complete removal of gluten from the diet. However, patients need to follow a strict gluten-free diet that results in symptomatic, serologic, and histologic remission in most patients. Histologic remission is usually complete in children, but recovery is slower and more frequently incomplete in adults. When remission has been achieved, yearly follow-up is recommended for adults, children, and adolescents. This article deals with conventional strategies used in order to follow-up patients on treatment and aiming to obtain the best clinical outcome.

Refractory celiac disease (RCD) refers to persistence of malnutrition and intestinal villus atrophy for more than 1 to 2 years despite strict gluten-free diet in patients with celiac disease. Diagnosis remains difficult and impacts treatment and follow-up. RCD has been subdivided into 2 subgroups according to the normal (RCDI) or abnormal phenotype of intraepithelial lymphocytes (IELs) (RCDII). RCDII is considered as a low-grade intraepithelial lymphoma and has a poor prognosis due to gastrointestinal and extraintestinal dissemination of the abnormal IELs, and high risk of overt lymphoma.

Celiac disease (CD) is an autoimmune enteropathy triggered by gluten. Gluten-free diets can be challenging because of their restrictive nature, inadvertent cross-contaminations, and the high cost of gluten-free food. Novel nondietary therapies are at the preclinical stage, clinical trial phase, or have already been developed for other indications and are now being applied to CD. These therapies include enzymatic gluten degradation, binding and sequestration of gluten, restoration of epithelial tight junction barrier function, inhibition of tissue transglutaminase–mediated potentiation of gliadin oligopeptide immunogenicity or of human leukocyte antigen–mediated gliadin presentation, induction of tolerance to gluten, and antiinflammatory interventions.

Non-celiac wheat sensitivity (NCWS) is characterized by gastrointestinal and extra-intestinal symptoms following the ingestion of gluten-containing cereals in subjects without celiac disease or wheat allergy. The identity of the molecular triggers in these cereals responsible for the symptoms of NCWS remains to be delineated. Recent research has identified a biological basis for the condition, with the observation of systemic immune activation in response to microbial translocation that appears to be linked to intestinal barrier defects. Ongoing research efforts are aimed at further characterizing the etiology, mechanism, and biomarkers of the condition.

GASTROENTEROLOGY
CLINICS OF NORTH AMERICA

THE CLINICS ARE AVAILABLE ONLINE!
Access your subscription at:
www.theclinics.com

Foreword

Celiac Disease, Gluten-Free, and Today's Fashionista

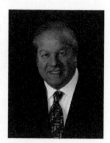

Alan L. Buchman, MD, MSPH, FACN, FACG, FACP, AGAF
Consulting Editor

First described by the famous ancient Greek physician Aretaeus of Cappadocia, "celiac" and the later-described "gluten-free" have become buzz words during this millennium. Individuals claim they feel much better when consuming a gluten-free diet. Is this gluten sensitivity? Is it a real disease entity? Rigorous studies have begun to investigate this in a scientific manor. A famous chef in Chicago once told me a number of years ago when restaurants were forced to come out with gluten-free menus that the same individuals who requested gluten-free meals were the same ones ordering bread pudding for dessert. "Gluten-free" has become a marketing call as great as, "Remember the Alamo." I'm sure gluten-free steak and potatoes are available, perhaps under the moniker, "Never had it, never will." Disease recognition is not always good for the disease and those it afflicts; the true facts often become distorted and diluted, although celiac disease likely continues to be underdiagnosed at the same time. In this issue of *Gastroenterology Clinics of North America*, Ben Lebwohl and Peter Green, two stalwarts in the field of celiac disease, have assembled an outstanding group of investigators who provide us with the latest facts about the disease, the breadth of the concern, and what we know about who it effects, why it affects them, how it affects them, and what effected individuals can do. We recognize now that the intestinal microbiome likely has a role in the development, and perhaps management, of celiac disease, perhaps through interaction with genetics. Celiac disease is a systemic disease that has been linked to extraintestinal organs as well as other autoimmune diseases. Although many investigational therapies have failed, others have shown promise as they advance to later-stage clinical trials. This is exciting

Gastroenterol Clin N Am 48 (2019) xiii–xiv
https://doi.org/10.1016/j.gtc.2018.10.002
0889-8553/19/© 2018 Published by Elsevier Inc.

news for the person who really does have celiac disease and really wants to eat that bread pudding.

Alan L. Buchman, MD, MSPH, FACN, FACG, FACP, AGAF
Intestinal Rehabilitation and Transplant Center
Department of Surgery
College of Medicine
The University of Illinois at Chicago
840 South Wood Street, Suite 402 Clinical Sciences Building, MC 958
Chicago, IL 60612, USA

Health Care Services Corporation
300 E. Randolph Street
Chicago, IL 60601, USA

E-mail address:
buchman@uic.edu

Preface

New Developments in Celiac Disease

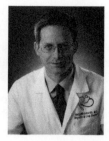 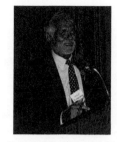

Benjamin Lebwohl, MD, MS   Peter H.R. Green, MD
Editors

The world of celiac disease is changing rapidly. From the mid-twentieth century forward, celiac disease was understood as an illness primarily affecting children, exclusively affecting the small intestine, and treated by life-long gluten restriction, with no other therapies on the horizon. In recent years, these aspects of celiac disease have been upended. This issue of *Gastroenterology Clinics of North America* documents the current state of understanding celiac disease during this time of major change.

The first portion of this collection features articles on the epidemiology of celiac disease, clinical features, aspects of diagnosis including histopathology, and a detailed description of the current treatment, the gluten-free diet. These articles cover the changing presentation of celiac disease, which is now recognized to develop de novo at any age, and the various systemic manifestations of this condition. The second portion of these articles discusses areas on the frontier of celiac disease research, including the rise in celiac disease incidence in Asia, studies of the interplay of celiac disease with the intestinal microbiome, and breakthroughs in the diagnosis and treatment of refractory celiac disease. An article on nondietary therapies for celiac disease covers a broad array of pharmacologic agents that are in various stages of development, including clinical trials. A concluding article focuses on nonceliac gluten sensitivity, an entity whose etiology and pathogenesis largely elude our understanding, but whose biology has begun to be studied with increasing scientific rigor.

We are grateful to the contributors of the articles comprising this issue, an international group of experts who have dedicated much time and effort to committing the latest in celiac disease research to the page. We would also like to thank Sara Watkins for her diligent editorial assistance and high standards when editing these articles. Most importantly, we acknowledge the irreplaceable contributions of our patients, who have volunteered to participate in research studies, shared their perspective and

Gastroenterol Clin N Am 48 (2019) xv–xvi
https://doi.org/10.1016/j.gtc.2018.10.001
0889-8553/19/© 2018 Published by Elsevier Inc.   **gastro.theclinics.com**

insights of living with celiac disease, and inspired us to spend our daily work in this scientific, medical, and ultimately humanistic venture.

Benjamin Lebwohl, MD, MS
The Celiac Disease Center at
Columbia University
180 Fort Washington Avenue, Suite 936
New York, NY 10032, USA

Peter H.R. Green, MD
Celiac Disease Center at
Columbia University
180 Fort Washington Avenue, Suite 936
New York, NY 10032, USA

E-mail addresses:
BL114@columbia.edu (B. Lebwohl)
PG11@columbia.edu (P.H.R. Green)

Epidemiology of Celiac Disease

Jonas F. Ludvigsson, MD, PhD[a,b,c,d,*], Joseph A. Murray, MD, PhD[e,f]

KEYWORDS

- Celiac disease • Epidemiology • Gluten • Incidence • Mortality • Prevalence
- Risk factors

KEY POINTS

- Celiac disease (CD) is a common chronic condition in many parts of the world.
- CD affects people of all ages, with a slight predisposition for women.
- The cause of CD requires both genetic and environmental factors, primarily and essentially the human leukocyte antigen types DQ2 or DQ8 and intake of gluten.
- CD has a broad range of presenting symptoms and syndromes that make detection challenging, with many patients remaining undiagnosed for long periods.
- Diagnosis relies on serology tests, although confirmation with intestinal biopsies is most often required.

INTRODUCTION

Celiac disease (CD) is an immune-mediated disease characterized by small intestinal inflammation, crypt hyperplasia, and villus atrophy.[1]

Disclosure: All authors have completed the ICMJE uniform disclosure form at www.icmje.org/coi_disclosure.pdf and declare that this project was supported by grants from the Swedish Society of Medicine and the Stockholm County Council, and the Swedish Research Council (grant 2013-2429).

Disclaimer: This article represents the views of the authors. The authors have nothing else to disclose.

[a] Department of Medical Epidemiology and Biostatistics, Karolinska Institutet, Solnavägen 1, Solna 171 77, Sweden; [b] Department of Pediatrics, Örebro University Hospital, Örebro, Sweden; [c] Division of Epidemiology and Public Health, School of Medicine, University of Nottingham, City Hospital, Clinical Sciences Building 2, Nottingham, UK; [d] Department of Medicine, Celiac Disease Center, Columbia University College of Physicians and Surgeons, New York, NY, USA; [e] Division of Gastroenterology and Hepatology, Department of Immunology, Mayo Clinic, 200 First Street Southwest, Rochester, MN 55905, USA; [f] University of Southern Denmark, Odense, Denmark

* Corresponding author. Department of Medical Epidemiology and Biostatistics, Karolinska Institutet, Solnavägen 1, Solna 171 77, Sweden.

E-mail address: jonasludvigsson@yahoo.com

Gastroenterol Clin N Am 48 (2019) 1–18
https://doi.org/10.1016/j.gtc.2018.09.004
0889-8553/19/© 2018 Elsevier Inc. All rights reserved.

Abbreviations	
CD	Celiac disease
CI	Confidence interval
HR	Hazard ratio
OR	Odds ratio

Methods

The authors used a PubMed search using the mesh terms "celiac disease" and "risk factors" up until March 1, 2018. This search identified 754 potentially relevant studies, the titles and abstracts of which were then reviewed by the lead author. These studies were then complemented with other studies known by the authors.

Aim

This article reviews risk factors for CD with a focus on environmental factors, its incidence and prevalence worldwide, and also mortality and other complications in CD.

Risk Factors

The literature on risk factors for CD is abundant, but most research has focused on childhood-onset CD. These days, CD is more often diagnosed in adulthood than In childhood.[2] Triggers of CD in adulthood may differ from those of childhood-onset CD.

CD may be present for many years before diagnosis, making insights into the triggering factors inherently more difficult to study in adults.[3] A summary of risk factors associated with CD is provided in **Table 1**.

Table 1
Factors associated with the development of celiac disease

Factor	Important	Weak or Uncertain
Gluten	Necessary for disease	—
Genetics	HLA DQ2or DQ8 is required Twin concordance Increased risk in disorders caused by chromosomal abnormalities	40 other genes with small additive effects Female sex
Infant nutrition	Gluten quantity	Breastfeeding reduces risk in children <2 y
Pregnancy and birth-related factors	Small for gestational age	Elective cesarean section (variable data) Season of birth Iron treatment in expectant mother
Place of living	Wheat growing, northern latitudes associated higher risk in United States	White
Infections and microbiome	Reovirus Infections Antibiotic exposure	Dysbiosis Poor oral health Influenza, lack of *Helicobacter* Rotavirus
Socioeconomic status and smoking	Smoking is negatively associated with celiac disease	High socioeconomic group No effect of smoking in pregnant mothers High maternal education level

Abbreviation: HLA, human leukocyte antigen.

Gluten

The first obvious risk factor in CD is gluten. People who are never exposed to gluten do not develop CD. The identification of a necessary cause sets CD apart from many other autoimmune diseases, such as type 1 diabetes and autoimmune thyroid disease, in which the triggering factors remain unknown. A large part of early risk factor research in CD has concentrated on infant nutrition. The main results of this research are discussed later.

Genetics

CD often occurs in families, having an 80% concordance rate in homozygous twins. The single most important genetic factors that drives risk are the class 2 human leukocyte antigen (HLA) genes. CD is strongly associated with certain common HLA types. DQ2 and DQ8, unlike other autoimmune diseases, are required for the disease to occur. The HLA genes also confer a gene dosage to risk. Individuals who have a double dose of DQ2 encoded by DQA1:0501 DQB1:0201 are 5 times more likely to have CD than individuals with just a single dose of DQ2. Almost all patients with CD carry DQ2 (90%), with approximately 5% to 7% carrying DQ8. A tiny proportion of patients have an alternative genetic type often incorporating half of the gene pair encoding DQ2; so-called DQ2.2. The latter is coded as DQA1:0501 DQB1:0201. The increased risk has been clearly shown in birth cohort studies as well as population studies in which HLA genetics are a primary driver for the risk of disease. However, most patients, even those with the highest HLA-determined genetic risk, never develop CD. Although HLA status is the predominant factor in the cause of CD,[4] it is not the only genetic factor. These genes alone are not sufficient for the disease to occur. Other factors, primarily gluten but also other genes, contribute to the risk of CD. It is estimated that the HLA-associated molecules contribute at least 40% of the heritable risk of CD. There are other genes in the other HLA region that contribute risk as well as at least 40 genes that are located outside of the major histocompatibility complex region that are linked to CD. However, the relative risk of each of these other non-HLA genes is small, only reaching significance in association studies incorporating many thousands of patients. Some of these genes encode proteins such as SH2B3. Evolutionary and functional analysis of celiac risk loci reveals SH2B3 as a protective factor against bacterial infection.[5] Others represent genes encoding long noncoding RNAs such as lnc13 RNA that may control expression of other genes often involved in the adaptive and innate immune systems.[6,7] In addition, genes related to mucosal integrity, epithelial function, and even metabolism are also associated with CD risk. Attempts have been made to combine HLA and non-HLA regions to generate a risk score. Studies on epigenetics, transcription regulation, and interaction between the host genome, the human genome, and the method genome relating to bacteria are ongoing and may provide further insights on the complex interaction between environmental factors and host genetics.

Several studies have also showed an increased risk of CD in patients with Down syndrome[8] and Turner syndrome.[9] Individuals with Down syndrome have higher interleukin-15 levels,[10] and interleukin is thought to be crucial for CD development.[11] Another risk factor for CD is female sex.[12] In several studies, about 60% of all patients with CD have been female.[13] At the same time, some studies indicate that women have more severe symptoms from CD than men,[14] and this may affect health-seeking behavior and ultimately the chance of being diagnosed. In contrast, a recent US study, in which more than 30,000 individuals from a single community were screened for CD, a more equal sex balance was found.[3,15] That health-seeking behavior in CD may differ by sex has also been noted in a recent US study, in which especially young men seemed less inclined to contact health care professionals for suspected CD.[16]

Infant nutrition

The natural starting point for any discussion about infant feeding and CD is the so-called Swedish epidemic.[17] Coinciding with a change in infant feeding recommendations, the incidence of CD in children aged less than 2 years increased from 50 to about 200 per 100,000 person-years between 1985 and 1987. The high incidence figures remained up until 1995 when they decreased equally dramatically to the original levels of around 50 per 100,000 person-years. This change in incidence, together with later studies suggesting either an increase[18–21] or on at least 1 occasion a decrease[22] in incidence argues that nongenetic factors play an important role for CD cause.

Clinical correlation Up until 2014, both age at gluten introduction and ongoing breast-feeding were regarded as near-established risk factors for CD.[23] However, with few exceptions,[24,25] studies on breastfeeding and CD have been based on retrospective data.[26–29] In the largest case-control study so far, the investigators found a lower risk of future CD in children aged less than 2 years at diagnosis but not in older children. The protective effect in young children was especially strong in those being breastfed beyond the introduction of gluten (odds ratio [OR], 0.36; 95% confidence interval [CI], 0.26–0.51). Two other studies[28,29] reported similar results; whereas a case-control study taking HLA status into account detected no association between breastfeeding at time of gluten introduction and CD. In contrast, another case-control study by Decker and colleagues[30] reported the opposite results. In that study, long breastfeeding was instead a positive risk factor for CD (OR, 1.99; 95% CI, 1.12–3.51).[30] Up until 2014, when the New England Journal of Medicine published the results of 2 landmark randomized clinical trials on infant feeding and CD,[31,32] there were 3 prospective studies on breastfeeding and CD. They all showed contradicting data, likely due of lack of statistical power. The US study by Norris and colleagues[24] observed 1560 children with HLA-DR3/DR4 through regular blood tests and questionnaires. Their main outcome measure was CD autoimmunity, which required either (1) 2 positive CD serology blood tests or (2) 1 positive blood test combined with a small intestinal biopsy consistent with CD. Some 49% (25 out of 51) of children with CD autoimmunity were breastfed when first introduced to wheat, barley, or rye compared with 44% (660 out of 1509) controls ($P > .05$; ie, no difference). Children with CD autoimmunity had a longer breastfeeding duration (median duration, 8.8 months) than controls (6.8 months).[24] In a Swedish study, Welander and colleagues[25] used prospectively collected data from the All Babies in Southeast Sweden (ABIS) study. This study found no association between breastfeeding duration and subsequent development of CD. Nor could they show any association between breastfeeding duration and later CD when taking age of gluten introduction, and prospectively recorded infections at time of gluten introduction, into account. However, there was a trend toward short breastfeeding as a protective factor against CD (eg, risk of later CD in offspring to mothers ending breastfeeding at 0–2 months of infant age: OR, 0.7; at 3–4 months, 0.7; and at 4–5 months, 0.3). None of these risk estimates were statistically significant.[25] In addition, the Oxford Record Linkage Study found similar cumulative incidences of CD among breastfed (32.4 out of 100,000) and nonbreastfed infants (43.2 out of 100,000) ($P = .28$). The exposure in the British study was "ever breastfed" and therefore cannot inform whether breastfeeding at time of gluten introduction protects against CD or not.

In 2014, Vriezinga and colleagues[31] and Lionetti and colleagues[32] independently reported a lack of association between age at gluten introduction, breastfeeding duration, and later CD. These randomized trials have been followed by at least 3 meta-analyses, either showing a small increased risk of CD (+25%) in children with a late introduction of gluten[33] or no association.[34] Instead, later research on gluten and risk of CD has focused on amount of gluten. Several studies have indicated that the differences in CD prevalence within Europe may be caused by different flour consumption patterns.[35–37]

However, several earlier studies were ecological (based on summary measures), and later research based on individual-based data has not been consistent. Although it has been hypothesized that large amounts of gluten early in life would be detrimental for the risk of CD, a recent article from The Environmental Determinants of Diabetes in the Young (TEDDY) study found that children with a low consumption at 6 months (and a large consumption later in life) were at the highest risk of CD.[38]

Recently, 2 studies explored other infant food exposures in CD. Hyytinen and colleagues[39] found no association between cow's milk consumption and CD and tissue transglutaminase levels, but this study may have been underpowered to rule out cow's milk as a risk factor for CD because the 95% CI for the main outcome measure ranged from 0.81 to 21.02. Data from the Generation R study in the Netherlands found a higher risk of CD autoimmunity in children with high intake of vegetables, vegetable oils, pasta, and grains and low consumption of refined cereals and sweet beverages at 1 year.[40] However, although the Generation R study is based on prospectively collected data for the food pattern, classification for the study of CD was made a posteriori.

In summarizing the literature so far, there is scarce evidence that age at gluten introduction, ongoing breastfeeding at gluten introduction, amount of gluten consumption, or other infant food patterns predispose to CD. However, gluten is a necessary cause for CD and earlier research does not rule out that gluten introduction or a certain amount of gluten, combined with other exposures, may trigger CD.

Pregnancy and birth-related factors
Given that infant CD typically debuts in the first year of life [OF] or shortly thereafter, it is natural to explore factors related to pregnancy and birth. At least 4 longitudinal cohort studies have contributed to this understanding: the Denver cohort, All Babies In southeast Sweden (ABIS) cohort, Norwegian Mother and Child Cohort Study (MoBa) cohort, and TEDDY cohort. Various studies have negated any association between maternal paracetamol consumption,[41] maternal antibiotics use,[41,42] maternal gluten consumption, and maternal and parental smoking.[43] It therefore seems that influences during pregnancy should, at the most, have a marginal impact on CD risk in offspring. One exception could be maternal iron supplementation during pregnancy.[44]

Maternal iron supplementation was linked to a +33% increased risk of CD in the offspring, whereas maternal anemia was not associated with future CD. Even if anemia per se was not linked to offspring CD in the Norwegian study, natural heredity patterns may explain the association with iron supplementation if pregnant women taking such supplements had lower hemoglobin levels than mothers without supplements. Many studies have found an increased prevalence of CD in iron-deficiency anemia[45,46] and, assuming that mothers with iron-supplements were more likely to have undiagnosed CD,[47] offspring may simply have inherited a greater tendency to develop CD, thereby explaining the 33% excess risk. However, Letner and colleagues[48] recently showed an association between total iron-binding capacity and CD, and the authors have previously found that hemochromatosis predicts later CD,[47] so a role for iron cannot be ruled out.

To our knowledge, the first study showing that small for gestational age in the newborn might be a risk factor for CD was that of Sandberg-Bennich and colleagues.[49] This finding was confirmed in the largest study so far, in which Marild and colleagues[50] compared 11,749 individuals with biopsy-verified CD and 53,887 age-matched and sex-matched controls. Small for gestational age was associated with a 1.21-fold increased risk of CD (95% CI, 1.09–1.35). Of note, 2 other studies have failed to detect any association,[51] and it remains uncertain whether fetal growth predisposes to CD. Marild and colleagues[50] also found a positive association with elective cesarean section (OR, 1.15; 95% CI, 1.04–1.26) but not with emergency cesarean section (OR, 1.02; 95% CI, 0.92–1.13). This finding is congruent with the hypothesis that the microbiota is abnormal and predisposes to CD only in children never in contact with the birth canal. A later Norwegian study[51] and the multinational TEDDY study[52] both refuted an association with cesarean section. Emilsson and colleagues[51] also examined elective cesarean section, whereas the TEDDY study did not.[52] The largest study to date combining the Norwegian and Danish mother baby cohorts showed no association with mode of delivery.[53] Meanwhile a smaller German study (N = 157 celiac cases) found an OR of 1.8 (95% CI, 1.13–2.88) for earlier cesarean section.[30] Recently, the authors also examined the influence of birthweight in 669 patients with CD with twins without CD.[54] Overall birth weight and future CD were not linked (OR per 1000-g increase in birth weight, 1.16; 95% CI, 0.97–1.38), but in male subjects we found a positive and statistically significant association (OR, 1.50; 95% CI, 1.11–2.02).[54]

In a sense, season of birth[55–57] can be thought of as a birth-related exposure. The largest of these studies on season[57] reported a 6% higher risk of future CD in children born during summer months. However, it was only through the magnitude of this study that such a small (potential) risk increase could be detected and, taken together, season-of-birth studies point toward an overall neutral relationship with CD.

In summary, pregnancy and birth-related factors are unlikely to play a major role in the development of CD.[58]

Place of living

It is evident that the prevalence of CD varies both between continents and between countries. The gradient between neighboring Sweden and Denmark, Finland and Estonia, and the low prevalence in Germany all point to the importance of environmental risk factors. Recently, one of us (J.A. Murray) found a strong gradient in CD in the United States, with a 5.4-fold higher risk of CD in those living north of the 40th degree compared with those living below the 30th degree.[59] Meanwhile, a north-south CD gradient (more in the south) has been shown in Sweden,[60] although it should be acknowledged that all of Sweden is above the 40th degree to begin with. Individuals on northern latitudes are more likely to have vitamin D deficiency, which was explored by Marild and colleagues.[61] This research group found no association between neonatal vitamin D levels and later CD. Among other vitamin levels examined in CD are vitamin A (isotretinoin). Vitamin A analogue use may be a risk factor for inflammatory bowel disease but has not been linked to CD.[62]

Infections and the microbiome

The first report of a potential infectious disease trigger in CD identified adenovirus as a possible culprit for CD.[63] Later on, Stene and Gale[64] suggested that prior rotavirus infections may predispose to CD. Note that the association between number of rotavirus infections and CD in that study was only statistically significant for trend analysis (P = .037). Comparing children without a rotavirus infection with those having 2 infections, the OR was not statistically significant (OR, 3.76; 95% CI, 0.76–18.7).[64] Another argument against rotavirus as a trigger of CD is the lack of decreased CD after the introduction of nationwide immunizations against this virus in several Nordic regions (personal communication, Ludvigsson, March 4, 2018). However, given the extensive comorbidity seen in CD.[125] reported a 1.8-fold increased risk of CD in children having an infection at time of gluten introduction, but the association failed to reach statistical significance (95% CI, 0.9–3.6). Even more interesting was the finding of a 2.6-fold increased risk of CD if this infection had been a gastroenteritis, but, because of few events, the 95% CI for this analysis was even wider (95% CI, 0.2–30.8). Also, Italian data have indicated a link between gastrointestinal infection and CD.[65]

A Norwegian study reported an association between frequent infections during the first year of life and CD,[66] although, of note, the association with gastroenteritis was not statistically significant. Röckert Tjernberg and colleagues[67] reported a statistically significantly increased risk for later CD in children with a prior hospital record of obstructive bronchitis, which, in small children, is almost exclusively caused by a viral infection. van Gils and colleagues[68] also recently reported an association between poor oral health and CD. In addition, Karhus and colleagues[69] reported a +29% increased risk of CD after both seasonal and H1N1 influenza. In that article, the investigators also noted an association between H1N1 influenza vaccination and CD, but that association was lower than for H1N1 infection per se.[69] Several earlier articles found that the H1N1 vaccination was associated with many autoimmune comorbidities, but these associations were seen both before and after vaccination,[70] and only for later narcolepsy has a causal relationship been established. When Myleus and colleagues[71] examined early childhood vaccinations and later CD they found no association.

A recent study suggested a role of a nonvirulent reovirus as potentially having a role in preventing tolerance to dietary antigens. Initially, using a mouse model, Bouziat and colleagues[72] showed that, when infection of a specific reovirus co-occurred with exposure to the introduction of either gluten or ovalbumin, tolerance to the dietary antigen was not achieved, likely through prevention of the formation of T-regulatory cells. Instead, the gut immune system developed a TH1 effector response. In addition, they showed that some patients with CD had increased levels of antireovirus antibodies. CD seemed to be associated with high titers to reovirus. Of course, questions remain as to whether this effect is specific to this particular reovirus or other viruses. The experimental work would support, in effect, a role for viral triggering in the initiation of an immune response to gluten, although its role in the perpetuation of inflammation and injury is as yet unexplored.[72]

The microbiome has been implicated in the cause of CD. An important role for the mucosally associated bacteria is to induce and maintain tolerance in the gut. Dysbiosis characterized by an altered ratio between relative abundances of Proteobacteria and lactobacilli has been described in untreated CD both in the stool and in the upper small intestine. Bacteria from the duodenum may alter the immune effect of gluten, with some decreasing and others increasing the immunogenicity of gluten-derived peptides.[73]

If the microbiome is involved in CD pathogenesis, this may also explain earlier findings of prevalent antibiotics use in patients with CD.[42,65] Both studies found a positive association with CD, and, consistent with this, the Italian study also reported a dose-response relationship.[65] Two other studies also indicating that the microbiome or the gastrointestinal micromilieu may be important to CD development are the articles by Lebwohl and colleagues.[74,75] In the first article, Lebwohl and colleagues[74] showed a strong inverse relationship between *Helicobacter pylori* colonization and risk of CD, and, in the second study, proton pump inhibitors (PPIs) were linked to a higher risk of CD.[75] It may be argued that such a link could be caused by confounding by indication (physicians prescribe PPIs for abdominal pain that is caused by undiagnosed CD). Although this cannot fully be excluded, the association with PPI remained[75] 1 year after prescription (OR, 2.28).

Not being part of the microbiome, vaccinations nevertheless influence the risk of infections and potentially later development of CD.

Socioeconomic status and smoking

In contrast with studies on cardiovascular disease, in which low socioeconomic status is often linked to disease, the opposite may be true for CD.[21,76] In Italy, high maternal education has also been linked to an increased risk of CD in the offspring.[65] However, the largest study so far in this field reported no substantial association between socioeconomic status and CD.[77]

Most earlier studies have reported a negative association between smoking and CD,[78–80] but there are exceptions,[81–83] and the largest study so far[82] has shown a positive association. Another form of tobacco, moist snuff use, has not been linked to CD.[83]

Other risk factors

Other risk factors that have been examined in relationship to CD include prior head trauma[84] and borrelia infection.[85]

The importance of genetics and environmental risk factors in Celiac disease It is clear from the current review that genetic risk factors are very important in CD, especially HLA. Assuming that, in a population in which everyone consumes gluten, earlier data based on the Swedish twin register (107,000 twins out of whom 513 had CD) suggest that, apart from HLA, non-HLA genetics explains 68% of the risk of CD and environmental factors explain 32% of the risk.[86]

Prevalence and Incidence

It is generally acknowledged that about 1% of the general population have CD,[1] whereas the proportion of diagnosed individuals varies between countries.[7] A high prevalence of CD was first noted in Sweden[1] and Finland[87] but, since the first reports, many studies have shown a prevalence around and more than 1%.[20,88] Higher prevalence figures have been shown in both younger[89] and older[90] populations. Prevalence rates around 1% have been shown not only in Europe but also in Asia.[91] Data from sub-Saharan Africa indicate substantially lower levels,[92] and CD seems rare among African Americans.[15]

As noted in **Fig. 1**, which shows a selection of relevant studies,[80,87,89,93–110] the prevalence of CD is generally higher when the diagnosis is based on serology than when a small intestinal biopsy is required for diagnosis.[111,112] Despite an increase in CD, there are still unexplained between-country differences in the prevalence of CD.[108]

The incidence of CD seems to be increasing,[18,20,88] even if a recent study suggests a stabilization (or even a decrease) of the CD incidence in Finland.[22]

Mortality in Celiac Disease

CD has been linked to many diseases in most organ systems, including circulation,[113–117] skin,[118,119] skeletal and osteoporosis,[120–122] digestive,[123,124] urinary,[125] respiratory,[126–130] endocrine,[113,131–134] lymphatic,[135] blood,[136] immune,[137] infectious

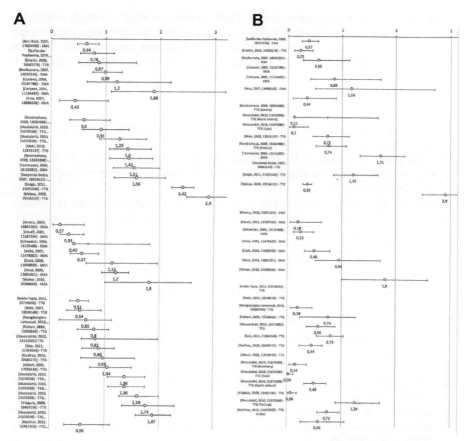

Fig. 1. (*A*) Seroprevalence of celiac disease in global populations (prevalence +95% CIs). (*B*) Biopsy-confirmed prevalence of celiac disease in global populations (±95% CIs). (*Data from* Refs.[80,87,89,93–110])

disease,[138] and nervous systems, which includes psychiatric disorders[139–146] (data on risk of stroke are inconsistent[147,148]).

It is important to underline that, with the exception of certain cardiovascular and respiratory diseases, absolute risks are low, and most patients with CD do not develop additional chronic diseases until old age.

However, given the extensive comorbidity seen in CD and the large number of associated disorders, the increased mortality in CD is expected. Earlier studies often reported highly increased risks of death,[149–152] but later studies[13,153] have shown lower risk estimates. When Tio and colleagues[154] reviewed the evidence up until 2012, they found a marginally increased risk of death (+29%). The 2 largest studies so far have shown a +39% increased risk[13] and no increased risk.[153] Among the explanations for the different findings of these two studies are between-country differences, including that smoking has been inversely linked to CD in the United Kingdom but not in Sweden. The studies are also based on different time periods.

The absolute mortality in the Swedish study was low and, for patients between 40 and 60 years of age with CD, 1 in 112 will die in the next year, compared with 1 in 159 individuals without a diagnosis of CD.[13] In the Swedish study, an increased risk of death was seen both in children and in adults, and throughout the study period (ie, also in recent years, when the importance of a gluten-free diet has been increasingly stressed). The most common cause of death in Swedish patients with CD was cardiovascular death, although the highest relative risks were seen for death from malignancy.

REFERENCES

1. Ludvigsson JF, Leffler DA, Bai JC, et al. The Oslo definitions for coeliac disease and related terms. Gut 2013;62(1):43–52.
2. Ludvigsson JF, Brandt L, Montgomery SM, et al. Validation study of villus atrophy and small intestinal inflammation in Swedish biopsy registers. BMC Gastroenterol 2009;9(1):19.
3. Choung RS, Larson SA, Khaleghi S, et al. Prevalence and morbidity of undiagnosed celiac disease from a community-based study. Gastroenterology 2017; 152(4):830–9.e5.
4. Liu E, Lee HS, Aronsson CA, et al. Risk of pediatric celiac disease according to HLA haplotype and country. N Engl J Med 2014;371(1):42–9.
5. Zhernakova A. Evolutionary and functional analysis of celiac risk loci reveals SH2B3 as a protective factor against bacterial infection. Am J Hum Genet 2010;86:970–7.
6. Castellanos-Rubio A, Santin I, Irastorza I, et al. TH17 (and TH1) signatures of intestinal biopsies of CD patients in response to gliadin. Autoimmunity 2009;42(1): 69–73.
7. Castellanos-Rubio A, Fernandez-Jimenez N, Kratchmarov R, et al. A long noncoding RNA associated with susceptibility to celiac disease. Science 2016; 352(6281):91–5.
8. Marild K, Stephansson O, Grahnquist L, et al. Down syndrome is associated with elevated risk of celiac disease: a nationwide case-control study. J Pediatr 2013;163(1):237–42.
9. Marild K, Stordal K, Hagman A, et al. Turner syndrome and celiac disease: a case-control study. Pediatrics 2016;137(2):e20152232.
10. Roat E, Prada N, Lugli E, et al. Homeostatic cytokines and expansion of regulatory T cells accompany thymic impairment in children with Down syndrome. Rejuvenation Res 2008;11(3):573–83.
11. Abadie V, Jabri B. IL-15: a central regulator of celiac disease immunopathology. Immunol Rev 2014;260(1):221–34.
12. Wingren CJ, Bjorck S, Lynch KF, et al. Coeliac disease in children: a social epidemiological study in Sweden. Acta Paediatr 2012;101(2):185–91.
13. Ludvigsson JF, Montgomery SM, Ekbom A, et al. Small-intestinal histopathology and mortality risk in celiac disease. JAMA 2009;302(11):1171–8.
14. Ciacci C, Cirillo M, Sollazzo R, et al. Gender and clinical presentation in adult celiac disease. Scand J Gastroenterol 1995;30(11):1077–81.
15. Choung RS, Ditah IC, Nadeau AM, et al. Trends and racial/ethnic disparities in gluten-sensitive problems in the United States: findings from the National Health and Nutrition Examination Surveys from 1988 to 2012. Am J Gastroenterol 2015; 110(3):455–61.
16. Dixit R, Lebwohl B, Ludvigsson JF, et al. Celiac disease is diagnosed less frequently in young adult males. Dig Dis Sci 2014;59(7):1509–12.
17. Ivarsson A, Persson LA, Nystrom L, et al. Epidemic of coeliac disease in Swedish children. Acta Paediatr 2000;89(2):165–71 [see comments].

18. Lohi S, Mustalahti K, Kaukinen K, et al. Increasing prevalence of coeliac disease over time. Aliment Pharmacol Ther 2007;26(9):1217–25.
19. Virta LJ, Kaukinen K, Collin P. Incidence and prevalence of diagnosed coeliac disease in Finland: results of effective case finding in adults. Scand J Gastroenterol 2009;44(8):933–8.
20. Ludvigsson JF, Rubio-Tapia A, van Dyke CT, et al. Increasing incidence of celiac disease in a North American population. Am J Gastroenterol 2013;108(5): 818–24.
21. Zingone F, West J, Crooks CJ, et al. Socioeconomic variation in the incidence of childhood coeliac disease in the UK. Arch Dis Child 2015;100(5):466–73.
22. Virta LJ, Saarinen MM, Kolho KL. Declining trend in the incidence of biopsy-verified coeliac disease in the adult population of Finland, 2005-2014. Aliment Pharmacol Ther 2017;46(11–12):1085–93.
23. Akobeng AK, Ramanan AV, Buchan I, et al. Effect of breast feeding on risk of coeliac disease: a systematic review and meta-analysis of observational studies. Arch Dis Child 2006;91(1):39–43.
24. Norris JM, Barriga K, Hoffenberg EJ, et al. Risk of celiac disease autoimmunity and timing of gluten introduction in the diet of infants at increased risk of disease. JAMA 2005;293(19):2343–51.
25. Welander A, Tjernberg AR, Montgomery SM, et al. Infectious disease and risk of later celiac disease in childhood. Pediatrics 2010;125(3):e530–6.
26. Auricchio S, Follo D, de Ritis G, et al. Does breast feeding protect against the development of clinical symptoms of celiac disease in children? J Pediatr Gastroenterol Nutr 1983;2(3):428–33.
27. Greco L, Auricchio S, Mayer M, et al. Case control study on nutritional risk factors in celiac disease. J Pediatr Gastroenterol Nutr 1988;7(3):395–9.
28. Falth-Magnusson K, Franzen L, Jansson G, et al. Infant feeding history shows distinct differences between Swedish celiac and reference children. Pediatr Allergy Immunol 1996;7(1):1–5.
29. Peters U, Schneeweiss S, Trautwein EA, et al. A case-control study of the effect of infant feeding on celiac disease. Ann Nutr Metab 2001;45(4):135–42.
30. Decker E, Engelmann G, Findeisen A, et al. Cesarean delivery is associated with celiac disease but not inflammatory bowel disease in children. Pediatrics 2010; 125(6):e1433–40.
31. Vriezinga SL, Auricchio R, Bravi E, et al. Randomized feeding intervention in infants at high risk for celiac disease. N Engl J Med 2014;371(14):1304–15.
32. Lionetti E, Castellaneta S, Francavilla R, et al. Introduction of gluten, HLA status, and the risk of celiac disease in children. N Engl J Med 2014;371(14):1295–303.
33. Pinto-Sanchez MI, Verdu EF, Liu E, et al. Gluten introduction to infant feeding and risk of celiac disease: systematic review and meta-analysis. J Pediatr 2016;168:132–43.e3.
34. Silano M, Agostoni C, Sanz Y, et al. Infant feeding and risk of developing celiac disease: a systematic review. BMJ Open 2016;6(1):e009163.
35. Michaelsen KF, Weile B, Larsen P, et al. Does the low intake of wheat in Danish infants cause the low incidence rate of coeliac disease? Acta Paediatr 1993; 82(6–7):605–6.
36. Weile B, Cavell B, Nivenius K, et al. Striking differences in the incidence of childhood celiac disease between Denmark and Sweden: a plausible explanation. J Pediatr Gastroenterol Nutr 1995;21(1):64–8.
37. Mitt K, Uibo O. Low cereal intake in Estonian infants: the possible explanation for the low frequency of coeliac disease in Estonia. Eur J Clin Nutr 1998;52(2):85–8.

38. Aronsson CA, Lee HS, Liu E, et al. Age at gluten introduction and risk of celiac disease. Pediatrics 2015;135(2):239–45.
39. Hyytinen M, Savilahti E, Virtanen SM, et al. Avoidance of cow's milk-based formula for at-risk infants does not reduce development of celiac disease: a randomized controlled trial. Gastroenterology 2017;153(4):961–70.e3.
40. Barroso M, Beth SA, Voortman T, et al. Dietary patterns after the weaning and lactation period are associated with celiac disease autoimmunity in children. Gastroenterology 2018;154(8):2087–96.e7.
41. Marild K, Kahrs CR, Tapia G, et al. Maternal infections, antibiotics, and paracetamol in pregnancy and offspring celiac disease: a cohort study. J Pediatr Gastroenterol Nutr 2017;64(5):730–6.
42. Marild K, Ludvigsson J, Sanz Y, et al. Antibiotic exposure in pregnancy and risk of coeliac disease in offspring: a cohort study. BMC Gastroenterol 2014;14:75.
43. Ludvigsson JF, Ludvigsson J. Parental smoking and risk of coeliac disease in offspring. Scand J Gastroenterol 2005;40(3):336–42.
44. Stordal K, Haugen M, Brantsaeter AL, et al. Association between maternal iron supplementation during pregnancy and risk of celiac disease in children. Clin Gastroenterol Hepatol 2014;12(4):624–31.e1-2.
45. Corazza GR, Valentini RA, Andreani ML, et al. Subclinical coeliac disease is a frequent cause of iron-deficiency anaemia. Scand J Gastroenterol 1995;30(2):153–6.
46. Mandal AK, Mehdi I, Munshi SK, et al. Value of routine duodenal biopsy in diagnosing coeliac disease in patients with iron deficiency anaemia. Postgrad Med J 2004;80(946):475–7.
47. Singh P, Arora S, Lal S, et al. Risk of celiac disease in the first- and second-degree relatives of patients with celiac disease: a systematic review and meta-analysis. Am J Gastroenterol 2015;110(11):1539–48.
48. Letner D, Peloquin J, Durand J, et al. Elevated total iron-binding capacity is associated with an increased risk of celiac disease. Dig Dis Sci 2015;60(12):3735–42.
49. Sandberg-Bennich S, Dahlquist G, Kallen B. Coeliac disease is associated with intrauterine growth and neonatal infections. Acta Paediatr 2002;91(1):30–3.
50. Marild K, Stephansson O, Montgomery S, et al. Pregnancy outcome and risk of celiac disease in offspring: a nationwide case-control study. Gastroenterology 2012;142(1):39–45.e3.
51. Emilsson L, Magnus MC, Stordal K. Perinatal risk factors for development of celiac disease in children, based on the prospective Norwegian Mother and Child Cohort Study. Clin Gastroenterol Hepatol 2015;13(5):921–7.
52. Koletzko S, Lee HS, Beyerlein A, et al. Cesarean section on the risk of celiac disease in the offspring: the teddy study. J Pediatr Gastroenterol Nutr 2018;66(3):417–24.
53. Dydensborg Sander S, Hansen AV, Stordal K, et al. Mode of delivery is not associated with celiac disease. Clin Epidemiol 2018;10:323–32.
54. Kuja-Halkola R, Lebwohl B, Halfvarson J, et al. Birth weight, sex, and celiac disease: a nationwide twin study. Clin Epidemiol 2017;9:567–77.
55. Kokkonen J, Simila S, Vuolukka P. The incidence of coeliac disease and pyloric stenosis in children in northern Finland. Ann Clin Res 1982;14(3):123–8.
56. Stene LC, Honeyman MC, Hoffenberg EJ, et al. Rotavirus infection frequency and risk of celiac disease autoimmunity in early childhood: a longitudinal study. Am J Gastroenterol 2006;101(10):2333–40.

57. Lebwohl B, Green PH, Murray JA, et al. Season of birth in a nationwide cohort of coeliac disease patients. Arch Dis Child 2013;98(1):48–51.
58. Marild K, Ludvigsson JF, Stordal K. Current evidence on whether perinatal risk factors influence coeliac disease is circumstantial. Acta Paediatr 2016;105(4): 366–75.
59. Unalp-Arida A, Ruhl CE, Choung RS, et al. Lower prevalence of celiac disease and gluten-related disorders in persons living in southern vs northern latitudes of the United States. Gastroenterology 2017;152(8):1922–32.e2.
60. Olsson C, Stenlund H, Hornell A, et al. Regional variation in celiac disease risk within Sweden revealed by the nationwide prospective incidence register. Acta Paediatr 2009;98(2):337–42.
61. Marild K, Tapia G, Haugen M, et al. Maternal and neonatal vitamin D status, genotype and childhood celiac disease. PLoS One 2017;12(7):e0179080.
62. Lebwohl B, Sundstrom A, Jabri B, et al. Isotretinoin use and celiac disease: a population-based cross-sectional study. Am J Clin Dermatol 2014;15(6):537–42.
63. Kagnoff MF, Paterson YJ, Kumar PJ, et al. Evidence for the role of a human intestinal adenovirus in the pathogenesis of coeliac disease. Gut 1987;28(8): 995–1001.
64. Stene LC, Gale EA. The prenatal environment and type 1 diabetes. Diabetologia 2013;56(9):1888–97.
65. Canova C, Zabeo V, Pitter G, et al. Association of maternal education, early infections, and antibiotic use with celiac disease: a population-based birth cohort study in northeastern Italy. Am J Epidemiol 2014;180(1):76–85.
66. Marild K, Kahrs CR, Tapia G, et al. Infections and risk of celiac disease in childhood: a prospective nationwide cohort study. Am J Gastroenterol 2015;110(10): 1475–84.
67. Röckert Tjernberg A, Bonnedahl J, Inghammar M, et al. Coeliac disease and invasive pneumococcal disease: a population-based cohort study. Epidemiol Infect 2017;145(6):1203–9.
68. van Gils T, Bouma G, Bontkes HJ, et al. Self-reported oral health and xerostomia in adult patients with celiac disease versus a comparison group. Oral Surg Oral Med Oral Pathol Oral Radiol 2017;124(2):152–6.
69. Karhus LL, Gunnes N, Stordal K, et al. Influenza and risk of later celiac disease: a cohort study of 2.6 million people. Scand J Gastroenterol 2018;53(1):15–23.
70. Bardage C, Persson I, Ortqvist A, et al. Neurological and autoimmune disorders after vaccination against pandemic influenza A (H1N1) with a monovalent adjuvanted vaccine: population based cohort study in Stockholm, Sweden. BMJ 2011;343:d5956.
71. Myleus A, Stenlund H, Hernell O, et al. Early vaccinations are not risk factors for celiac disease. Pediatrics 2012;130(1):e63–70.
72. Bouziat R, Hinterleitner R, Brown JJ, et al. Reovirus infection triggers inflammatory responses to dietary antigens and development of celiac disease. Science 2017;356(6333):44–50.
73. Caminero A, Galipeau HJ, McCarville JL, et al. Duodenal bacteria from patients with celiac disease and healthy subjects distinctly affect gluten breakdown and immunogenicity. Gastroenterology 2016;151(4):670–83.
74. Lebwohl B, Blaser MJ, Ludvigsson JF, et al. Decreased risk of celiac disease in patients with *Helicobacter pylori* colonization. Am J Epidemiol 2013;178(12): 1721–30.
75. Lebwohl B, Spechler SJ, Wang TC, et al. Use of proton pump inhibitors and subsequent risk of celiac disease. Dig Liver Dis 2014;46(1):36–40.

76. Namatovu F, Stromgren M, Ivarsson A, et al. Neighborhood conditions and celiac disease risk among children in Sweden. Scand J Public Health 2014;42(7): 572–80.
77. Olen O, Bihagen E, Rasmussen F, et al. Socioeconomic position and education in patients with coeliac disease. Dig Liver Dis 2012;44(6):471–6.
78. Vazquez H, Smecuol E, Flores D, et al. Relation between cigarette smoking and celiac disease: evidence from a case-control study. Am J Gastroenterol 2001; 96(3):798–802.
79. Snook JA, Dwyer L, Lee-Elliott C, et al. Adult coeliac disease and cigarette smoking. Gut 1996;39(1):60–2 [see comments].
80. West J, Logan RF, Hill PG, et al. Seroprevalence, correlates, and characteristics of undetected coeliac disease in England. Gut 2003;52(7):960–5.
81. Patel AH, Loftus EV Jr, Murray JA, et al. Cigarette smoking and celiac sprue: a case-control study. Am J Gastroenterol 2001;96(8):2388–91.
82. Ludvigsson JF, Montgomery SM, Ekbom A. Smoking and celiac disease: a population-based cohort study. Clin Gastroenterol Hepatol 2005;3(9):869–74.
83. Ludvigsson JF, Nordenvall C, Jarvholm B. Smoking, use of moist snuff and risk of celiac disease: a prospective study. BMC Gastroenterol 2014;14:120.
84. Ludvigsson JF, Hadjivassiliou M. Can head trauma trigger celiac disease? Nation-wide case-control study. BMC Neurol 2013;13:105.
85. Alaedini A, Lebwohl B, Wormser GP, et al. *Borrelia* infection and risk of celiac disease. BMC Med 2017;15(1):169.
86. Kuja-Halkola R, Lebwohl B, Halfvarson J, et al. Heritability of non-HLA genetics in coeliac disease: a population-based study in 107 000 twins. Gut 2016;65(11): 1793–8.
87. Maki M, Mustalahti K, Kokkonen J, et al. Prevalence of celiac disease among children in Finland. N Engl J Med 2003;348(25):2517–24.
88. West J, Fleming KM, Tata LJ, et al. Incidence and prevalence of celiac disease and dermatitis herpetiformis in the UK over two decades: population-based study. Am J Gastroenterol 2014;109(5):757–68.
89. Myleus A, Ivarsson A, Webb C, et al. Celiac disease revealed in 3% of Swedish 12-year-olds born during an epidemic. J Pediatr Gastroenterol Nutr 2009;49(2): 170–6.
90. Vilppula A, Kaukinen K, Luostarinen L, et al. Increasing prevalence and high incidence of celiac disease in elderly people: a population-based study. BMC Gastroenterol 2009;9:49.
91. Singh P, Arora S, Singh A, et al. Prevalence of celiac disease in Asia: a systematic review and meta-analysis. J Gastroenterol Hepatol 2016;31(6):1095–101.
92. Cataldo F, Lio D, Simpore J, et al. Consumption of wheat foodstuffs not a risk for celiac disease occurrence in Burkina Faso. J Pediatr Gastroenterol Nutr 2002; 35(2):233–4.
93. Szaflarska-Poplawska A, Parzecka M, Muller L, et al. Screening for celiac disease in Poland. Med Sci Monit 2009;15(3):PH7–11.
94. Castano L, Blarduni E, Ortiz L, et al. Prospective population screening for celiac disease: high prevalence in the first 3 years of life. J Pediatr Gastroenterol Nutr 2004;39(1):80–4.
95. Carlsson AK, Axelsson IE, Borulf SK, et al. Serological screening for celiac disease in healthy 2.5-year-old children in Sweden. Pediatrics 2001;107(1):42–5.
96. Kondrashova A, Mustalahti K, Kaukinen K, et al. Lower economic status and inferior hygienic environment may protect against celiac disease. Ann Med 2008;40(3):223–31.

97. Korponay-Szabo IR, Szabados K, Pusztai J, et al. Population screening for coeliac disease in primary care by district nurses using a rapid antibody test: diagnostic accuracy and feasibility study. BMJ 2007;335(7632):1244–7.
98. Dalgic B, Sari S, Basturk B, et al. Prevalence of celiac disease in healthy Turkish school children. Am J Gastroenterol 2011;106(8):1512–7.
99. Riestra S, Fernandez E, Rodrigo L, et al. Prevalence of coeliac disease in the general population of northern Spain. Strategies of serologic screening. Scand J Gastroenterol 2000;35(4):398–402.
100. Hovell CJ, Collett JA, Vautier G, et al. High prevalence of coeliac disease in a population-based study from Western Australia: a case for screening? Med J Aust 2001;175(5):247–50.
101. Schweizer JJ, von Blomberg BM, Bueno-de Mesquita HB, et al. Coeliac disease in The Netherlands. Scand J Gastroenterol 2004;39(4):359–64.
102. Volta U, Bellentani S, Bianchi FB, et al. High prevalence of celiac disease in Italian general population. Dig Dis Sci 2001;46(7):1500–5.
103. Walker MM, Murray JA, Ronkainen J, et al. Detection of celiac disease and lymphocytic enteropathy by parallel serology and histopathology in a population-based study. Gastroenterology 2010;139(1):112–9.
104. Rubio-Tapia A, Herman ML, Ludvigsson JF, et al. Severe spruelike enteropathy associated with olmesartan. Mayo Clin Proc 2012;87(8):732–8.
105. Roka V, Potamianos SP, Kapsoritakis AN, et al. Prevalence of coeliac disease in the adult population of central Greece. Eur J Gastroenterol Hepatol 2007;19(11):982–7.
106. Alessandrini S, Giacomoni E, Muccioli F. Mass population screening for celiac disease in children: the experience in Republic of San Marino from 1993 to 2009. Ital J Pediatr 2013;39:67.
107. Godfrey JD, Brantner TL, Brinjikji W, et al. Morbidity and mortality among older individuals with undiagnosed celiac disease. Gastroenterology 2010;139(3):763–9.
108. Mustalahti K, Catassi C, Reunanen A, et al. The prevalence of celiac disease in Europe: results of a centralized, international mass screening project. Ann Med 2010;42(8):587–95.
109. Vilppula A, Collin P, Maki M, et al. Undetected coeliac disease in the elderly: a biopsy-proven population-based study. Dig Liver Dis 2008;40(10):809–13.
110. Kochhar R, Sachdev S, Kochhar R, et al. Prevalence of celiac disease in healthy blood donors: a study from north India. Dig Liver Dis 2012;44(6):530–2.
111. Dube C, Rostom A, Sy R, et al. The prevalence of celiac disease in average-risk and at-risk Western European populations: a systematic review. Gastroenterology 2005;128(4 Suppl 1):S57–67.
112. Kang JY, Kang AH, Green A, et al. Systematic review: worldwide variation in the frequency of coeliac disease and changes over time. Aliment Pharmacol Ther 2013;38(3):226–45.
113. Emilsson L, Andersson B, Elfstrom P, et al. Risk of idiopathic dilated cardiomyopathy in 29 000 patients with celiac disease. J Am Heart Assoc 2012;1(3):e001594.
114. Ludvigsson JF, James S, Askling J, et al. Nationwide cohort study of risk of ischemic heart disease in patients with celiac disease. Circulation 2011;123(5):483–90.
115. Emilsson L, Carlsson R, Holmqvist M, et al. The characterisation and risk factors of ischaemic heart disease in patients with coeliac disease. Aliment Pharmacol Ther 2013;37(9):905–14.

116. Emilsson L, Smith JG, West J, et al. Increased risk of atrial fibrillation in patients with coeliac disease: a nationwide cohort study. Eur Heart J 2011;32(19): 2430–7.

117. Elfstrom P, Hamsten A, Montgomery SM, et al. Cardiomyopathy, pericarditis and myocarditis in a population-based cohort of inpatients with coeliac disease. J Intern Med 2007;262(5):545–54.

118. Ludvigsson JF, Rubio-Tapia A, Chowdhary V, et al. Increased risk of systemic lupus erythematosus in 29,000 patients with biopsy-verified celiac disease. J Rheumatol 2012;39(10):1964–70.

119. Ludvigsson JF, Lindelof B, Rashtak S, et al. Does urticaria risk increase in patients with celiac disease? A large population-based cohort study. Eur J Dermatol 2013;23(5):681–7.

120. Vestergaard P, Mosekilde L. Fracture risk in patients with celiac disease, Crohn's disease, and ulcerative colitis: a nationwide follow-up study of 16,416 patients in Denmark. Am J Epidemiol 2002;156(1):1–10.

121. Zanchetta MB, Longobardi V, Costa F, et al. Impaired bone microarchitecture improves after one year on gluten-free diet: a prospective longitudinal HRpQCT study in women with celiac disease. J Bone Miner Res 2017;32(1):135–42.

122. Ludvigsson JF, Michaelsson K, Ekbom A, et al. Coeliac disease and the risk of fractures - a general population-based cohort study. Aliment Pharmacol Ther 2007;25(3):273–85.

123. Sadr-Azodi O, Sanders DS, Murray JA, et al. Patients with celiac disease have an increased risk for pancreatitis. Clin Gastroenterol Hepatol 2012;10(10): 1136–42.e3.

124. Leffler DA, Kelly CP. Celiac disease and gastroesophageal reflux disease: yet another presentation for a clinical chameleon. Clin Gastroenterol Hepatol 2011;9(3):192–3.

125. Welander A, Prutz KG, Fored M, et al. Increased risk of end-stage renal disease in individuals with coeliac disease. Gut 2012;61(1):64–8.

126. Ludvigsson JF, Wahlstrom J, Grunewald J, et al. Coeliac disease and risk of sarcoidosis. Sarcoidosis Vasc Diffuse Lung Dis 2007;24(2):121–6.

127. Ludvigsson JF, Hemminki K, Wahlstrom J, et al. Celiac disease confers a 1.6-fold increased risk of asthma: a nationwide population-based cohort study. J Allergy Clin Immunol 2011;127(4):1071–3.

128. Ludvigsson JF, Inghammar M, Ekberg M, et al. A nationwide cohort study of the risk of chronic obstructive pulmonary disease in coeliac disease. J Intern Med 2012;271(5):481–9.

129. Zingone F, Abdul Sultan A, Crooks CJ, et al. The risk of community-acquired pneumonia among 9803 patients with coeliac disease compared to the general population: a cohort study. Aliment Pharmacol Ther 2016;44(1):57–67.

130. Ludvigsson JF, Sanders DS, Maeurer M, et al. Risk of tuberculosis in a large sample of patients with coeliac disease–a nationwide cohort study. Aliment Pharmacol Ther 2011;33(6):689–96.

131. Kaukinen K, Halme L, Collin P, et al. Celiac disease in patients with severe liver disease: gluten-free diet may reverse hepatic failure. Gastroenterology 2002; 122(4):881–8.

132. Elfstrom P, Sundstrom J, Ludvigsson JF. Systematic review with meta-analysis: associations between coeliac disease and type 1 diabetes. Aliment Pharmacol Ther 2014;40(10):1123–32.

133. Elfstrom P, Montgomery SM, Kampe O, et al. Risk of thyroid disease in individuals with celiac disease. J Clin Endocrinol Metab 2008;93(10):3915–21.

134. Elfstrom P, Montgomery SM, Kampe O, et al. Risk of primary adrenal insufficiency in patients with celiac disease. J Clin Endocrinol Metab 2007;92(9):
3595–8.
135. Elfstrom P, Granath F, Ekstrom Smedby K, et al. Risk of lymphoproliferative malignancy in relation to small intestinal histopathology among patients with celiac
disease. J Natl Cancer Inst 2011;103(5):436–44.
136. Olen O, Montgomery SM, Elinder G, et al. Increased risk of immune thrombocy-
topenic purpura among inpatients with coeliac disease. Scand J Gastroenterol
2008;43(4):416–22.
137. Ludvigsson JF, Olen O, Bell M, et al. Coeliac disease and risk of sepsis. Gut
2008;57(8):1074–80.
138. Marild K, Fredlund H, Ludvigsson JF. Increased risk of hospital admission for
influenza in patients with celiac disease: a nationwide cohort study in Sweden.
Am J Gastroenterol 2010;105(11):2465–73.
139. Hadjivassiliou M, Grunewald RA, Kandler RH, et al. Neuropathy associated with
gluten sensitivity. J Neurol Neurosurg Psychiatry 2006;77(11):1262–6.
140. Hadjivassiliou M, Grunewald R, Sharrack B, et al. Gluten ataxia in perspective:
epidemiology, genetic susceptibility and clinical characteristics. Brain 2003;
126(Pt 3):685–91.
141. Ludvigsson JF, Reutfors J, Osby U, et al. Coeliac disease and risk of mood
disorders–a general population-based cohort study. J Affect Disord 2007;
99(1–3):117–26.
142. Mollazadegan K, Kugelberg M, Lindblad BE, et al. Increased risk of cataract
among 28,000 patients with celiac disease. Am J Epidemiol 2011;174(2):
195–202.
143. Ludvigsson JF, Zingone F, Tomson T, et al. Increased risk of epilepsy in biopsy-
verified celiac disease: a population-based cohort study. Neurology 2012;
78(18):1401–7.
144. Ludvigsson JF, Sellgren C, Runeson B, et al. Increased suicide risk in coeliac
disease–A Swedish nationwide cohort study. Dig Liver Dis 2011;43(8):616–22.
145. Butwicka A, Lichtenstein P, Frisen L, et al. Celiac disease is associated with
childhood psychiatric disorders: a population-based study. J Pediatr 2017;
184:87–93.e1.
146. Marild K, Stordal K, Bulik CM, et al. Celiac disease and anorexia nervosa: a
nationwide study. Pediatrics 2017;139(5) [pii:e20164367].
147. West J, Logan RF, Card TR, et al. Risk of vascular disease in adults with diagnosed coeliac disease: a population-based study. Aliment Pharmacol Ther
2004;20(1):73–9.
148. Ludvigsson JF, West J, Card T, et al. Risk of stroke in 28,000 patients with celiac
disease: a nationwide cohort study in Sweden. J Stroke Cerebrovasc Dis 2012;
21(8):860–7.
149. West J, Logan RF, Smith CJ, et al. Malignancy and mortality in people with
coeliac disease: population based cohort study. BMJ 2004;329(7468):716–9.
150. Grainge MJ, West J, Card TR, et al. Causes of death in people with celiac disease spanning the pre- and post-serology era: a population-based cohort study
from Derby, UK. Am J Gastroenterol 2011;106(5):933–9.
151. Peters U, Askling J, Gridley G, et al. Causes of death in patients with celiac disease in a population-based Swedish cohort. Arch Intern Med 2003;163(13):
1566–72.
152. Corrao G, Corazza GR, Bagnardi V, et al. Mortality in patients with coeliac disease and their relatives: a cohort study. Lancet 2001;358(9279):356–61.

153. Abdul Sultan A, Crooks CJ, Card T, et al. Causes of death in people with coeliac disease in England compared with the general population: a competing risk analysis. Gut 2015;64(8):1220–6.
154. Tio M, Cox MR, Eslick GD. Meta-analysis: coeliac disease and the risk of all-cause mortality, any malignancy and lymphoid malignancy. Aliment Pharmacol Ther 2012;35(5):540–51.

Celiac Disease
Clinical Features and Diagnosis

Isabel A. Hujoel, MD[a,1], Norelle R. Reilly, MD[b,1],
Alberto Rubio-Tapia, MD[a,*]

KEYWORDS

- Celiac disease • Celiac sprue • Diagnosis • Clinical presentation • Symptoms

KEY POINTS

- The presentation of celiac disease in adults and children is changing, with an increase in nonclassical symptoms.
- Case finding is the recommended modality to identify undiagnosed cases of celiac disease; however, there is increasing evidence that it may not be effective.
- Screening for celiac disease should be performed with serology.
- Although European pediatric guidelines recommend a serology-based diagnosis in some cases, biopsy is still recommended in diagnosis for adults.

Although virtually an unknown condition in the mid-20th century, celiac disease has since increased in both recognition and frequency.[1] The seroprevalence of celiac disease is currently approximately 1% in European[2] and US[3] populations, although the majority of these individuals have not been diagnosed.[2,4] Although the gap between undiagnosed and recognized cases may be narrowing,[4] the challenge of early diagnosis remains in both children and adults.

CELIAC DISEASE PRESENTATION
Clinical Features in the Adult Population

Celiac disease is now increasingly recognized in the adult and geriatric populations and presents with a spectrum of symptoms and associated conditions.[5] In 2013, the Oslo definitions were published, suggesting terms to classify these varied clinical presentations.[6] Celiac disease is now recognized to present as symptomatic disease, which includes gastrointestinal and extraintestinal manifestations, and subclinical

Disclosure Statement: No financial disclosures to declare.
[a] Division of Gastroenterology and Hepatology, Mayo Clinic, 200 1st Street Southwest, Rochester, MN 55905, USA; [b] Division of Pediatric Gastroenterology, Columbia University Medicine Center, 630 West 168th Street, PH-17, New York, NY 10032, USA
[1] Isabel A. Hujoel and Norelle R. Reilly are co-first authors.
* Corresponding author.
E-mail address: rubiotapia.alberto@mayo.edu

Gastroenterol Clin N Am 48 (2019) 19–37
https://doi.org/10.1016/j.gtc.2018.09.001
0889-8553/19/© 2018 Elsevier Inc. All rights reserved.

disease, which refers to cases that do not have symptoms and signs to trigger clinical suspicion for the disease.[6] Symptomatic celiac disease can be further divided into classical and nonclassical celiac disease. Any case with malabsorption is defined as classical disease and all other cases as nonclassical.

The presentation of diagnosed celiac disease has been changing, with a shift toward older individuals with more mild disease.[5] This change has been attributed to increased awareness, better diagnostics, earlier detection through serologic testing, and environmental factors such as increased wheat consumption.[5,7] Symptomatic, classical disease was previously the most common presentation, and although it remains a prominent mode of presentation, subclinical and nonclassical cases now make up roughly 30% and 40% to 60% of new cases, respectively.[5,8] The demographics of newly diagnosed cases seem to be changing as well, with an increase in the median age at diagnosis to the third and fourth decades, although the elevated female to male ratio, estimated at roughly 3:1, has remained stable over time.[5,8] The distribution of body mass index among newly diagnosed patients has also increased, with an estimated 40% presenting as overweight/obese at diagnosis.[5]

Presentation also seems to vary between sexes and ages, with females typically diagnosed at a younger age and presenting more frequently with constipation, bloating, and iron deficiency anemia.[5,9] Additionally, females and the elderly tend to have more associated autoimmune conditions than their male and younger counterparts.[5,10] The incidence of celiac disease diagnosed in those over age 65 has been increasing, with elderly men being diagnosed more frequently than elderly women. The most common symptom in this age group is anemia, and micronutrient deficiencies may be the only presenting feature. Gastrointestinal symptoms are less prevalent in the elderly and, if present, tend to be mild.[10]

More than one-half of adults will have gastrointestinal symptoms and weight loss at presentation.[8,9] Diarrhea remains the most common gastrointestinal symptom at presentation, although it has been significantly decreasing in frequency over time.[5] In order of decreasing frequency, other gastrointestinal symptoms include bloating, aphthous stomatitis, alternating bowel habits, constipation, and gastroesophageal reflux disease.[8] Less common gastrointestinal symptoms include persistent vomiting and chronic abdominal pain. However, gastrointestinal symptoms are common in the general population and there is poor correlation between the presence of common gastrointestinal symptoms and undiagnosed celiac disease.[11]

Celiac disease can affect almost any organ system, which leads to numerous extraintestinal symptoms that are present in roughly one-half to two-thirds of cases, and that some studies suggest may be more prevalent than gastrointestinal symptoms[5,8] (Table 1). The most common extraintestinal symptoms in order of frequency have been identified as osteoporosis, anemia (most commonly secondary to iron deficiency), celiac hepatitis, and recurrent miscarriages.[8]

Autoimmune conditions can be found in 35% of patients of celiac disease, and individuals with celiac disease are more likely to have more than 1 autoimmune disease.[12] Hashimoto's thyroiditis is the most commonly associated autoimmune disorder, found in roughly 20% to 30% of patients; however, its frequency in celiac disease has been decreasing over time.[5,8,12] Of adults with autoimmune thyroid disease, 2.7% have celiac disease and celiac disease is more common in hyperthyroidism than hypothyroidism.[13] Psoriasis is the second most commonly associated autoimmune condition (4.3%) followed by type 1 diabetes mellitus, which is found in roughly 4% of cases of celiac disease (6% of adults with type 1 diabetes mellitus have celiac disease), and Sjogren's syndrome (2.4%).[5,8,12,14]

Table 1
Extraintestinal manifestations of celiac disease

	Demographics/Prevalence	Pathophysiology	Treatment	Notes
Hematologic				
Anemia	Common (20%–30%)[8,9,71] Adults > children Common in elderly	Most commonly secondary to iron deficiency (which may be due to malabsorption and occult bleeding)[72] Vitamin B$_{12}$ and Folate deficiency also are common Anemia of chronic disease[71]	Nutritional supplementation	Macrocytic anemia uncommon[71] Possible sign of more severe disease[73] Up to ~9% of iron deficiency anemia may be due to celiac disease[74] Lack of response to intravenous iron supplementation is a clue to underlying celiac disease[75]
Hyposplenism	Common (19%–80%)[76] More common when autoimmune conditions present	Hemodynamic changes Reticular–endothelial dysfunction	Pneumococcal vaccinations	Increased risk for infections, specifically by encapsulated bacteria such as pneumococcus[77]
Other hematologic findings: IgA deficiency(1.9%),[8] low cholesterol, thromboctosis, thrombocytopenia, leukopenia, venous thromboembolism, lymphoma (particularly intestinal)[72]				
Musculoskeletal				
Osteoporosis	Common (10%–50%)[8,9]	Malabsorption ↑ Cytokines Autoimmune	Gluten-free diet Calcium and vitamin D supplementation	Worse in cases with gastrointestinal symptoms Unclear if ↑ fracture risk Test for celiac disease in those with osteoporosis of unclear cause
Arthritis/arthralgia	Common (22%–30%)[78]	Autoimmune	Gluten-free diet	Both axial and peripheral
Other: fibromyalgia-like symptoms (2.2%)[8]				

(continued on next page)

Table 1
(continued)

	Demographics/ Prevalence	Pathophysiology	Treatment	Notes
Skin				
Dermatitis herpetiformis	Common (4%–20%)[8,79] More common in men Typically younger individuals (15–40)	Autoimmune (antibody deposition in skin)	Gluten-free diet Symptomatic treatment: dapsone, sulphapyridine[80]	Recovery after initiation of gluten-free diet can take months Considered pathognomonic for celiac disease Typically gastrointestinal symptoms are absent
Oral findings				
Aphthous ulcers	Common (18%–25%)[8,81]	Unknown	Gluten-free diet	
Dental enamel hypoplasias	Common (50% of cases of celiac disease)[82]	Immune mediated Nutritional deficiencies	None	Could be only manifestation of celiac disease Develops in those who have celiac disease during tooth mineralization (<7 y old)
Other oral findings: geographic tongue				
Neurologic				
Gluten ataxia	Rare May have slight male predominance Onset commonly during middle age[83]	Autoimmune (antibody deposition in brain tissue)	In patients with cerebellar ataxia, celiac disease antibodies, and no other diagnosis → trial gluten-free diet (response suggests gluten ataxia diagnosis)[75]	Can have either slow onset or be rapidly progressive Gastrointestinal symptoms rare[83] Presents with cerebellar ataxia Damage cannot be reversed, so early diagnosis is crucial
Peripheral neuropathy	Common (≤30%)[84]	Unknown: thought to be related to autoimmunity or inflammation	Gluten-free diet	If not treated quickly, may have permanent damage

Epilepsy	Rare	Unknown	Gluten-free diet[85]	~6% of epileptics may have celiac disease[85] People with celiac disease have 2.7-fold increased risk of epilepsy[86] May be associated with cerebral calcifications
Headache	Common (5%–46%)[8,84]	Unknown: postulated that ↑ proinflammatory cytokines leads to vascular tone disorder	Gluten-free diet	Includes migraine, tension, and mixed headaches
Other neurologic/psychiatric symptoms: schizophrenia,[87] dysthymia,[84] chronic fatigue				
Cardiopulmonary				
Lane-Hamilton syndrome	Rare[88]	Autoimmune	Supportive Gluten-free diet	Celiac disease presenting with pulmonary hemosiderosis Fewer than one-half the cases have gastrointestinal symptoms[88]
Gastrointestinal system (excluding luminal)				
Hypertransaminasemia ("celiac hepatitis")	Common (≤40% of adults)[89]	Increased intestinal permeability and inflammation Malnutrition Bacterial dysbiosis[90]	Gluten-free diet (normalization in 6–12 mo)	Celiac disease present in up to 9% of people with unexplained hypertransaminesemia[91] Mild nonspecific histologic changes on liver biopsy
Pancreatitis (acute and chronic)	Acute pancreatitis → uncommon Chronic pancreatitis → common among those undergoing endoscopic ultrasound (26%)[92]	Duodenal inflammation causing recurrent sphincter of Oddi obstruction	Sphincterotomy	People with celiac disease have a 3-fold increased risk of pancreatitis[93]

(continued on next page)

Table 1
(continued)

	Demographics/ Prevalence	Pathophysiology	Treatment	Notes
Pancreatic exocrine insufficiency	Common (estimates range from 4%–80%)[94]	Loss of intestinal brush border proteins Low cholecystokinin levels	Gluten-free diet Pancreatic enzyme replacement therapy	Common cause of persistent diarrhea in those with celiac disease on gluten-free diet
Other less commonly associated liver conditions: autoimmune hepatitis, autoimmune cholangitis, primary biliary cirrhosis, primary sclerosing cholangitis, vital hepatitis, fatty liver, nonalcoholic steatohepatitis, severe cryptogenic hepatopathy[90] People with celiac disease are 2–6 times more likely to develop liver disease, and people with liver disease are 4–6 times more likely to develop celiac disease				
Reproductive				
Infertility[95] Miscarriage[95] Intrauterine growth restriction[95] Preterm delivery[95] Low birth weight[95]	Common	Nutrient deficiency (ie zinc, selenium, folic acid) Autoimmune	Gluten-free diet significantly reduces risk	Test women with unexplained infertility, recurrent miscarriage, and intrauterine growth restriction for celiac disease (an up to 8-fold increased risk of having celiac disease) Often no other symptoms of celiac disease Higher risk in untreated patients than treated[95]

Other reproductive symptoms: delayed menarche; early menopause; amenorrhea; shorter duration of time when fertile (improved with gluten-free diet); short breastfeeding period (improved with gluten-free diet)[95]; decreased ovarian reserve[96]

Other conditions associated with celiac disease include connective tissue disorders, several genetic conditions, as well as inflammatory bowel disease. Commonly associated connective tissue disorders include Sjogren's syndrome and systemic sclerosis (1.7%).[8] Celiac disease is also more prevalent in Down syndrome (5.8%),[15] Turner syndrome, and William syndrome. Inflammatory bowel disease has a higher prevalence in the celiac disease cohort as compared with the general population, and in 1 study was estimated at 3%.[16]

Although celiac disease is increasing in incidence, most cases remain undiagnosed. A recent case-control study found that this undiagnosed population has a similar frequency of classical and extraintestinal symptoms as the general population, and in fact is less likely to have chronic diarrhea and dyspepsia.[17] The undiagnosed population is more likely to have hypothyroidism, and over time to develop osteoporosis, autoimmune conditions, chronic fatigue, and thyroiditis. It may be that the undiagnosed population is asymptomatic or that their symptoms are too mild to rise to clinical attention; regardless, a large proportions of the undiagnosed population seems to be clinically silent.

Clinical Features in Children

As in adult populations, over time there has been an evolution in disease presentation in children.[18] Early literature pertaining to celiac disease or "sprue" characterized the condition as one marked by wasting and steatorrhea.[19,20] Before the recognition of gluten as a key component to disease pathogenesis, mortality was observed to be as high as 36% in children.[21]

Although celiac disease is no longer viewed as a lethal condition of childhood, the classic presentation of celiac disease as a malabsorptive and stunting syndrome of early childhood has been noted to be predominant even as recently as 30 years ago,[22] and remains a common mode of presentation for very young children (infants or preschool age).[23] Very young children may also be more likely to have total villus atrophy on small bowel biopsy.[24]

Despite some features remaining consist with time, there has more generally been a shift in pediatric disease presentations of celiac disease, with children now diagnosed more commonly at an older age and with less frequent classical or gastrointestinal complaints.[25,26] Abdominal pain is now a common mode of presentation in children.[18] Extraintestinal manifestations of celiac disease may include oral aphthous ulcerations or other oral manifestations, such as dental enamel defects.[27] Headaches, arthralgias or arthritis, and nutritional deficits including iron deficiency anemia and bone fragility may prompt diagnosis.

In recent years, some investigators have noted less variability in disease presentation in children, suggesting a plateau in these observed shifts.[28] The gradual change in celiac disease presentation has been attributed at least in part to an evolution of available serologic testing methods enabling disease recognition in more subtle or asymptomatic cases.[29,30] Cases of children diagnosed owing to screening, many asymptomatic, have become more common with time.[18,31] Relatives of individuals with celiac disease are at increased risk of developing this condition and may be diagnosed owing to screening in the absence of clear symptoms.[31,32] Those with IgA deficiency are both at greater risk of developing celiac disease, and also pose a diagnostic challenge given the lack of sensitivity of tissue transglutaminase (tTG) antibody for diagnosing these individuals.[33] Other associated conditions, such as type 1 diabetes and trisomy 21, may also prompt serologic screening given the increased prevalence of celiac disease in these populations.

DIAGNOSIS OF CELIAC DISEASE IN CHILDREN AND ADULTS

The diagnosis of celiac disease relies on clinical features and serologic and histologic findings (**Fig. 1**). The current guidelines for diagnosis of celiac disease in adults and children recommend case finding, which involves screening populations felt to be at high risk for the disease owing to associated symptoms, signs, conditions, or family history.[34–36] However, there is increasing evidence to suggest that this method may not be effective.[17] Although there are some proponents for mass screening, the US Preventive Services Task Force recently released a statement against testing for celiac disease in asymptomatic individuals owing to the lack of evidence showing benefit.[37] Although more effective methods are needed to identify who should be tested for celiac disease, case finding remains the recommended strategy.

Given the invasive nature and expense of endoscopy and biopsy, serologic testing is used as a screening test for celiac disease. The original antibodies were targeted against native gliadin; however, owing to low sensitivity and specificity, testing for these antibodies has since been abandoned. Since then, more specific and sensitive antibodies have been discovered, targeted against endomysium (EMA) and tTG as well as against synthetic deamidated gliadin peptides (DGP). Although the guidelines differ, tTG-IgA is the most commonly recommended screening test owing to its reported high sensitivity (**Table 2**). However, there is increasing concern that the true sensitivity of this test may be lower than previously estimated. Sequential testing with tTG-IgA and EMA or DGP-IgG, the latter combination being recommended by the British Society of Gastroenterology, may be more sensitive screening tests.[35] Point-of-care tests are now available; however, further data are needed on their diagnostic accuracy.[38]

Diagnosis in the Adult Population

In the adult population, endoscopy with small intestinal biopsy remains the gold standard and is required for diagnosis. There are several endoscopic findings that suggest celiac disease, such as a mosaic tile pattern, prominent submucosal capillary fissures, loss of circular folds, and scalloping; however, these findings are not sensitive and their absence should not affect the decision to biopsy (**Fig. 2**).[39] Chromoendoscopy may highlight mucosal changes, although 1 study estimated that one-third of newly diagnosed cases of celiac disease had a normal endoscopic appearance.[40] The majority of cases of celiac disease will have patchy mucosal changes, with more significant injury in the proximal intestine. Additionally, roughly 10% of cases will only have mucosal changes in the duodenal bulb. It is therefore crucial for endoscopists to collect 4 to 6 biopsy specimens from the duodenum including 1 or 2 biopsies from the duodenal bulb, and to note the location that the specimens were collected to increase the diagnostic yield.[41] A single biopsy collected per pass has been recommended to improve orientation.[42] However, adherence to these recommendations is low in clinical practice and studies suggest significant variability in performance between endoscopists, likely stemming from insufficient specimens, failure to biopsy the duodenal bulb, or failure to biopsy at all.[41]

The characteristic histologic changes consistent with celiac disease involve the superficial small intestinal mucosa and include increased intraepithelial lymphocytes, crypt elongation (also called hyperplasia or hypertrophy), and loss of villus height in the form of partial or complete villus atrophy (**Fig. 3**). The lamina propria often has an infiltrate of plasma and lymphocytic cells. The increased intraepithelial lymphocytes tend to localize in the tips of villi and are predominantly CD8[+] T cells; this characteristic is often quantified as the lymphocyte count per 100 enterocytes. The degree of

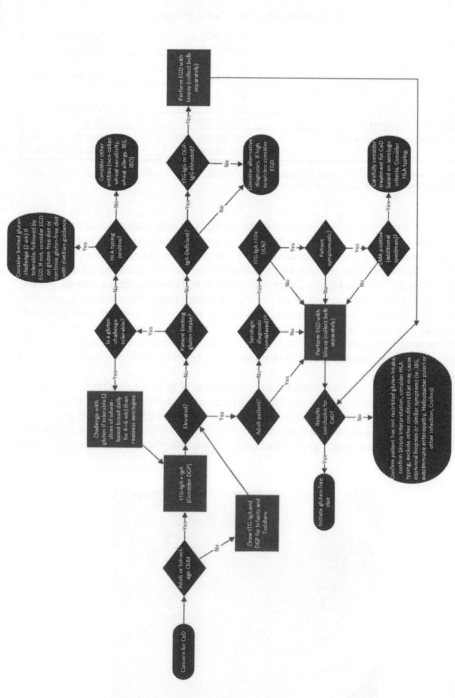

Fig. 1. An algorithm to approach the diagnosis of celiac disease (CeD). [a] A serologic diagnosis for a child should be considered carefully and in the context of local guidelines and laboratory standards. Even among children technically fulfilling criteria for a serologic diagnosis, this method may not be appropriate in all cases. DGP, deamidated gliadin peptides; EGD, esophagogastroduodenoscopy; EMA, endomysium; IBD, inflammatory bowel disease; IBS, irritable bowel syndrome; tTG, tissue transglutaminase; ULN, upper limit of normal.

Table 2
Sensitivities and specificities of serologic testing in celiac disease

	Sensitivity (Range), %	Specificity (Range), %
Antigliadin antibody	IgA: 85 (57–100) IgG: 85 (42–100)	IgA: 90 (47–94) IgG: 80 (50–94)
Antideamidated gliadin peptide	IgA: 88 (74–100) IgG: 80 (63–95)	IgA: 95 (90–99) IgG: 98 (90–99)
Endomysial antibody	95 (86–100)	99 (97–100)
Antitissue transglutaminase	IgA: 98 (78–100) IgG: 70 (45–95)	IgA: 98 (90–100) IgG: 95 (94–100)

Adapted from Leffler D, Schuppan D. Update on serologic testing in celiac disease. Am J Gastroenterol 2010;105(12):2523; with permission.

alteration of the villus architecture and crypt elongation may also be described as the ratio of the villus height to crypt depth, with decreasing values indicating greater histologic change. Two grading schemes have been developed to classify, trend, and compare histologic changes: the Marsh-Oberhuber and the Corazza-Villanacci systems **(Table 3)**.[43,44] The Marsh-Oberhuber system is more qualitative and subjective than the Corazza-Villanacci system and may have less concordance among pathologists.[45] Studies suggest that these 2 systems are rarely used in practice and, when they are, there is poor agreement between pathologists in grading, although not in respect to the presence or absence of disease. Perhaps because of these limitations, there has been a movement in research toward more quantitative scoring mechanisms.[46]

It is important to counsel patients on consuming a gluten-containing diet before serologic and/or histologic testing. The amount of daily gluten intake and the duration of time required to avoid false-negative testing is not clear. Classically, 10 g of gluten per day for 6 to 8 weeks was recommended. However, more recent data suggest that a shorter course of at least 3 g/d for 2 weeks may be effective in the majority of adults

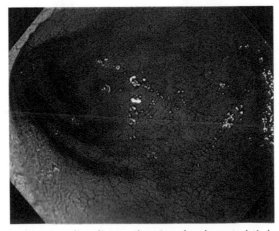

Fig. 2. Endoscopy findings in celiac disease showing the characteristic loss of circular folds, fissuring, and cobblestone appearance of the duodenal mucosa.

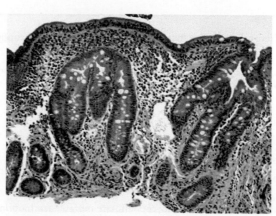

Fig. 3. Characteristic histologic findings in celiac disease. This specimen shows total villus atrophy, increased intraepithelial lymphocytes (80 intraepithelial lymphocytes per 100 epithelial cells), and crypt hyperplasia (stain: hematoxylin and eosin; original magnification ×40).

with celiac disease.[34,47] If a patient is already on a gluten-free diet, baseline serologic testing should be obtained. If this is negative, HLA typing can be performed to check for permissive genetics. If positive, a gluten challenge can be performed.

Clinicians may be faced with individuals who have villus atrophy on duodenal biopsy but negative serology. These cases can represent either an alternative disease process or seronegative celiac disease (**Box 1**). The tTG antibodies have been found in

Table 3
Marsh-Oberhuber and Corazza-Villanacci systems for classification of small bowel histology

Marsh-Oberhuber System	Villus Architecture	Crypts	Intraepithelial Lymphocytosis	Corazza-Villanacci System
0	Normal	Normal	None	
I (infiltrative)	Normal	Normal	Increased[a]	Grade A (nonatrophic)
II (hyperplastic)	Normal	Enlarged, increased division[b]	Increased	
IIIa (partial villus atrophy)	Short, blunt villi[b]	Enlarged[b]	Increased	Grade B1 (atrophic)
IIIb (subtotal villus atrophy)	Atrophic[b]	Enlarged,[b] increased immature epithelial cells	Increased	
IIIc (hypoplastic)	Total atrophy, complete loss of villi	Severe hyperplasia	Increased	Grade B2 (atrophic)

[a] The threshold for the Corazza-Villanacci system of 25 intraepithelial lymphocytes per 100 enterocytes, and for the Marsh-Oberhuber system of 40 intraepithelial lymphocytes per 100 enterocytes.
[b] The ratio of villus height to crypt depth of <3:1 to meet grade B1 criteria in the Corazza-Villanacci system (no thresholds for the Marsh-Oberhuber system).
Data from Oberhuber G. Histopathology of celiac disease. Biomed Pharmacother 2000;54(7):368–72; and Corazza G, Villanacci V. Coeliac disease: some considerations on the histological diagnosis. J Clin Path 2005;58:573–4.

Box 1
Conditions aside from celiac disease that can lead to duodenal villus atrophy

Infections[a]
  Whipple disease, infectious enteritis, tuberculosis, human immunodeficiency virus infection, *Helicobacter pylori*, *Giardia*

Tropical sprue[a]

Small-bowel bacterial overgrowth[a]

Common variable immunodeficiency-associated enteropathy

Autoimmune enteropathy

Collagenous sprue

Medication-associated enteropathy[a]
  Nonsteroidal antiinflammatory drugs, mycophenolate mofetil, azathioprine, olmesartan (and potentially other angiotensin-receptor blocker medications)

Intestinal lymphoma

Eosinophilic enteritis

Crohn's disease

Amyloidosis

Peptic duodenitis[a]

Malnutrition

Ischemia

Radiation enteritis

  [a] More commonly seen in practice.

---

the small bowel mucosa of seronegative cases, leading to the hypothesis that these antibodies are unable to pass into the circulation. This finding, along with the clinical features identified in case-series, suggests that seronegative celiac disease may represent more severe disease.[48] Diagnosis of seronegative celiac disease requires exclusion of alternative causes of villus atrophy, response to a gluten-free diet, and permissive HLA typing.

The converse situation, with positive serology and a normal biopsy, or increased intraepithelial lymphocytes with no atrophy, may also be seen, and may represent either potential celiac disease or a false-positive test result. HLA typing to rule out celiac disease if negative and/or a trial of a gluten-free diet can be considered to further characterize these cases.

Serologic Testing in Children: Special Considerations

For most IgA-sufficient children beyond the toddler years, the tTG-IgA antibody is the diagnostic tool of choice to detect celiac disease,[49–51] demonstrating a sensitive and specific diagnostic tool with a sensitivity and specificity of 90% or greater.[52] It should be remembered that occasionally results may vary when tests from different manufacturers are used, however.[53] EMA-IgA antibody performs similarly in terms of sensitivity (≥90%), although its specificity is even greater (98.2%),[52] which may be useful in groups such as those with autoimmune conditions such as type 1 diabetes, where tTG-IgA may sometimes lack specificity.[54] Although EMA may serve as an acceptable first-line screening tool in low-risk populations,[55] greater cost and user-dependent accuracy make tTG-IgA preferable in most populations.

For infants and young children with suspected celiac disease, especially those less than 2 years of age, tTG-IgA or DGP antibodies are recommended.[56] DGP-IgA has a sensitivity ranging between 80.7% and 95.1% (specificity, 86.3%–93.1%) and DGP-IgG has a sensitivity of 80.1% to 98.6% (specificity, 86.0%–96.9%).[52] DGP, particularly IgG, has demonstrated comparable sensitivity to tTG-IgA in young school-aged children (<7 years), although this sensitivity may diminish for older children.[57,58] In very young children, the sensitivity of DGP-IgG antibody may be superior to tTG[59] and to DGP-IgA antibody,[60] although other studies suggest that tTG-IgA alone is comparable[49] or superior to[61] both DGP-IgG and DGP-IgA in children younger than 2 years. Most societies recommend tTG-IgA in addition to DGP antibodies when celiac disease is suspected in a child less than age 2 years.[50]

Immunoglobulin A Deficiency

The level of IgA alters the sensitivity of IgA-based serologies. IgA levels tend to be lower among the youngest children and increase with age, with adult levels present by approximately age 6 to 7 years.[62] IgA levels may also be low in those with selective IgA deficiency. Although IgA antibodies are used typically, in cases of IgA deficiency, IgG antibodies should be used. Either IgG antibody to DGP or tTG may be used, although the sensitivity of tTG-IgG may be slightly superior.[63] In isolation in general population use, however, the specificity of tTG-IgG is poor[64] and generally a low positive tTG titer in a patient who is IgA sufficient should be regarded as a false-positive result.

Confirmatory Testing for Celiac Disease in Children

Recommendations as to how to proceed after abnormal serologic testing for celiac disease in children differs by geographic region. In North America, guidelines for the management of children with suspected celiac disease recommend proceeding to a small bowel biopsy for confirmation of the diagnosis before exclusion or limitation of gluten from the child's diet.[51,65] A separate biopsy collected from the duodenal bulb has been recommended in children as in adults, given variability in mucosal lesions of celiac disease in young patients.[66]

In 2012, guidelines from the European Society for Pediatric Gastroenterology, Hepatology, and Nutrition provided for a serologically based diagnosis of celiac disease in select cases of symptomatic children with a tTG-IgA level greater than 10 times the upper limit of normal for the laboratory, who additionally had a confirmatory positive EMA IgA antibody collected separately.[50] These guidelines seem to function well in practice among European populations,[67] and although some have suggested similar outcomes when these guidelines were applied to North American populations,[68] others have not.[69] Applying this guidance to groups outside of Europe may be acceptable, although a deeper understanding of local laboratories is warranted before reliably doing so given the heterogeneity in assays used.[68,70]

Human Leukocyte Antigen Typing

HLA typing has usefulness as a rule-out test in celiac disease owing to the high negative predictive value. Risk genes for celiac disease include HLA DQ2 (DQA1*05:01/05:05 and DQB1*02:01/02:02) and HLA DQ8 (DQA1*03:01 and DQB1*03:02). The presence of either HLA DQ2 or DQ8 is pivotal in the pathogenesis of celiac disease and therefore their absence indicates that development of celiac disease is extremely unlikely. These haplotypes are prevalent in the community (30%–40% of Caucasian population); however, only a small percentage of individuals with those haplotypes have celiac disease (3%). Therefore, HLA typing is beneficial in ruling out celiac disease, but cannot be used for diagnosis. The identification of a risk gene for celiac disease has been suggested for those diagnosed based on serologies alone.[50] However, the value of HLA typing in symptomatic patients with elevated tTG antibody more than 10 times the upper limit of normal and subsequent positive EMA antibody in a separate serum sample is controversial. HLA typing has also been recommended as a screening measure for seronegative first-degree relatives of an individual with celiac disease to determine the usefulness of ongoing serologic screening,[50,65] as well as for those with a mismatch between serologic and histologic findings.[50] Although the absence of a risk gene effectively rules out a diagnosis of celiac disease, it is important to recognize the capability of the performing laboratory to identify HLA DQ2 heterodimers as individual carriage of one-half of the DQ2 molecule, particularly of DQB1*02, still confers risk of celiac disease.

REFERENCES

1. Rubio-Tapia A, Kyle RA, Kaplan EL, et al. Increased prevalence and mortality in undiagnosed celiac disease. Gastroenterology 2009;137(1):88–93.
2. Mustalahti K, Catassi C, Reunanen A, et al. The prevalence of celiac disease in Europe: results of a centralized, international mass screening project. Ann Med 2010;42(8):587–95.
3. Rubio-Tapia A, Ludvigsson JF, Brantner TL, et al. The prevalence of celiac disease in the United States. Am J Gastroenterol 2012;107(10):1538–44 [quiz: 1537, 1545].
4. Choung RS, Unalp-Arida A, Ruhl CE, et al. Less hidden celiac disease but increased gluten avoidance without a diagnosis in the United States: findings from the national health and nutrition examination surveys from 2009 to 2014. Mayo Clin Proc 2017;92(1):30–8.
5. Dominguez Castro P, Harkin G, Hussey M, et al. Changes in presentation of celiac disease in Ireland from the 1960s to 2015. Clin Gastroenterol Hepatol 2017; 15(6):864–71.
6. Ludvigsson JF, Leffler DA, Bai J, et al. The Oslo definitions for coeliac disease and related terms. Gut 2013;62(1):43–52.
7. Ramakrishna B, Makharia G, Chetri K, et al. Prevalence of adult celiac disease in India: regional variations and associations. Am J Gastroenterol 2016;111(1): 115–23.
8. Volta U, Caio G, Stanghellini V, et al. The changing clinical profile of celiac disease: a 15-year experience (1988-2012) in an Italian referral center. BMC Gastroenterol 2014;14:194.
9. Schosler L, Christensen L, Hvas C. Symptoms and findings in adult-onset celiac disease in a historical Danish patient cohort. Scand J Gastroenterol 2016;51(3): 288–94.
10. Kalkan C, Karakaya F, Soykan I. Similarities and differences between older and young adult patients with celiac disease. Geriatr Gerontol Int 2017;17(11):2060–7.
11. Choung R, Rubio-Tapia A, Lahr B, et al. Evidence against routine testing of patients with functional gastrointestinal disorders for celiac disease: a population-based study. Clin Gastroenterol Hepatol 2015;13(11):1937–43.
12. Bibbo S, Pes G, Usai-Satta P, et al. Chronic autoimmune disorders are increased in coeliac disease: a case-control study. Medicine (Baltimore) 2017;96(47): e8562.

13. Roy A, Laszkowska M, Sundstrom J, et al. Prevalence of celiac disease in patients with autoimmune thyroid disease: a meta-analysis. Thyroid 2016;26(7): 880–90.
14. Elfstrom P, Sundstrom J, Ludvigsson J. Systematic review with meta-analysis: associations between coeliac disease and type 1 diabetes. Aliment Pharmacol Ther 2014;40(10):1123–32.
15. Du Y, Shan L, Cao Z, et al. Prevalence of celiac disease in patients with Down syndrome: a meta-analysis. Oncotarget 2017;9(4):5387–96.
16. Kocsis D, Toth Z, Csontos A, et al. Prevalence of inflammatory bowel disease among coeliac disease patients in a Hungarian coeliac centre. BMC Gastroenterol 2015;15:141.
17. Hujoel I, Van Dyke C, Brantner T, et al. Natural history and clinical detection of undiagnosed celiac disease in a North American community. Aliment Pharmacol Ther 2018;47(10):1358–66.
18. Almallouhi E, King KS, Patel B, et al. Increasing incidence and altered presentation in a population-based study of pediatric celiac disease in North America. J Pediatr Gastroenterol Nutr 2017;65(4):432–7.
19. Miller R. A note on gluteal wasting as a sign of Coeliac disease. Arch Dis Child 1927;2(9):189–90.
20. Howell CA. An early sign in sprue; the split-unsplit fat ratio in the faeces. Lancet 1947;2(6463):55.
21. Hardwick C. Prognosis in coeliac disease: a review of seventy-three cases. Arch Dis Child 1939;14(80):279–94.
22. George EK, Mearin ML, Franken HC, et al. Twenty years of childhood coeliac disease in The Netherlands: a rapidly increasing incidence? Gut 1997;40(1):61–6.
23. Tapsas D, Hollen E, Stenhammar L, et al. The clinical presentation of coeliac disease in 1030 Swedish children: changing features over the past four decades. Dig Liver Dis 2016;48(1):16–22.
24. Tanpowpong P, Broder-Fingert S, Katz AJ, et al. Age-related patterns in clinical presentations and gluten-related issues among children and adolescents with celiac disease. Clin Transl Gastroenterol 2012;3:e9.
25. Steens RF, Csizmadia CG, George EK, et al. A national prospective study on childhood celiac disease in the Netherlands 1993-2000: an increasing recognition and a changing clinical picture. J Pediatr 2005;147(2):239–43.
26. Roma E, Panayiotou J, Karantana H, et al. Changing pattern in the clinical presentation of pediatric celiac disease: a 30-year study. Digestion 2009;80(3): 185–91.
27. Ferraz EG, Campos Ede J, Sarmento VA, et al. The oral manifestations of celiac disease: information for the pediatric dentist. Pediatr Dent 2012;34(7):485–8.
28. Kivela L, Kaukinen K, Lahdeaho ML, et al. Presentation of celiac disease in Finnish children is no longer changing: a 50-year perspective. J Pediatr 2015; 167(5):1109–15.e1.
29. McGowan KE, Castiglione DA, Butzner JD. The changing face of childhood celiac disease in North America: impact of serological testing. Pediatrics 2009; 124(6):1572–8.
30. Garnier-Lengline H, Brousse N, Candon S, et al. Have serological tests changed the face of childhood coeliac disease? A retrospective cohort study. BMJ Open 2012;2(6) [pii:e001385].
31. Fasano A, Berti I, Gerarduzzi T, et al. Prevalence of celiac disease in at-risk and not-at-risk groups in the United States: a large multicenter study. Arch Intern Med 2003;163(3):286–92.

32. Bardella MT, Elli L, Velio P, et al. Silent celiac disease is frequent in the siblings of newly diagnosed celiac patients. Digestion 2007;75(4):182–7.
33. Meini A, Pillan NM, Villanacci V, et al. Prevalence and diagnosis of celiac disease in IgA-deficient children. Ann Allergy Asthma Immunol 1996;77(4):333–6.
34. Rubio-Tapia A, Hill I, Kelly C, et al. American College of Gastroenterology Clinical Guideline: diagnosis and management of celiac disease. Am J Gastroenterol 2013;108(5):656–77.
35. Ludvigsson J, Bai J, Biagi F, et al. Diagnosis and management of adult coeliac disease: guidelines from the British Society of Gastroenterology. Gut 2014;63: 1210–28.
36. Bai J, Ciacci C. World Gastroenterology Organisation global guidelines: celiac disease February 2017. J Clin Gastroenterol 2017;51(9):755–68.
37. Bibbins-Domingo K, Grossman D, Curry S, et al. Screening for celiac disease: US Preventive Services Task Force Recommendation Statement. JAMA 2017; 317(12):1252–7.
38. Lau M, Sanders D. Optimizing the diagnosis of celiac disease. Curr Opin Gastroenterol 2017;33(3):173–80.
39. Barada K, Habib R, Malli A, et al. Prediction of celiac disease at endoscopy. Endoscopy 2014;46(2):110–9.
40. Niveloni S, Fiorini A, Dezi R, et al. Videoduodenoscopy and vital dye staining as indicators of mucosal atrophy of celiac disease. Gastrointest Endosc 1998;47(3): 223–9.
41. Lebwohl B, Kapel R, Neugut A, et al. Adherence to biopsy guidelines increases celiac disease diagnosis. Gastrointest Endosc 2011;74(1):103–9.
42. Latorre M, Lagana SM, Freedberg DE, et al. Endoscopic biopsy technique in the diagnosis of celiac disease: one bite or two? Gastrointest Endosc 2015;81(5): 1228–33.
43. Oberhuber G. Histopathology of celiac disease. Biomed Pharmacother 2000; 54(7):368–72.
44. Corazza G, Villanacci V. Coeliac disease: some considerations on the histological diagnosis. J Clin Pathol 2005;58:573–4.
45. Corazza G, Villanacci V, Zambelli C, et al. Comparison of the interobserver reproducibility with different histologic criteria used in celiac disease. Clin Gastroenterol Hepatol 2007;5(7):838–43.
46. Adelman D, Murray J, Wu T, et al. Measuring change in small intestinal histology in patients with celiac disease. Am J Gastroenterol 2018;113(3):339–47.
47. Leffler D, Schuppan D, Pallav K, et al. Kinetics of the histological, serological and symptomatic responses to gluten challenge in adults with coeliac disease. Gut 2013;62(7):996–1004.
48. Salmi T, Collin P, Korponay-Szabo I, et al. Endomysial antibody-negative coeliac disease: clinical characteristics and intestinal autoantibody deposits. Gut 2006; 55(12):1746–53.
49. Basso D, Guariso G, Fogar P, et al. Antibodies against synthetic deamidated gliadin peptides for celiac disease diagnosis and follow-up in children. Clin Chem 2009;55(1):150–7.
50. Husby S, Koletzko S, Korponay-Szabo IR, et al. European Society for Pediatric Gastroenterology, Hepatology, and Nutrition guidelines for the diagnosis of coeliac disease. J Pediatr Gastroenterol Nutr 2012;54(1):136–60.
51. Hill ID, Dirks MH, Liptak GS, et al. Guideline for the diagnosis and treatment of celiac disease in children: recommendations of the North American Society for

Pediatric Gastroenterology, Hepatology and Nutrition. J Pediatr Gastroenterol Nutr 2005;40(1):1–19.

52. Giersiepen K, Lelgemann M, Stuhldreher N, et al. Accuracy of diagnostic antibody tests for coeliac disease in children: summary of an evidence report. J Pediatr Gastroenterol Nutr 2012;54(2):229–41.

53. Van Meensel B, Hiele M, Hoffman I, et al. Diagnostic accuracy of ten second-generation (human) tissue transglutaminase antibody assays in celiac disease. Clin Chem 2004;50(11):2125–35.

54. Lewis NR, Scott BB. Systematic review: the use of serology to exclude or diagnose coeliac disease (a comparison of the endomysial and tissue transglutaminase antibody tests). Aliment Pharmacol Ther 2006;24(1):47–54.

55. Harewood GC, Murray JA. Diagnostic approach to a patient with suspected celiac disease: a cost analysis. Dig Dis Sci 2001;46(11):2510–4.

56. Amarri S, Alvisi P, De Giorgio R, et al. Antibodies to deamidated gliadin peptides: an accurate predictor of coeliac disease in infancy. J Clin Immunol 2013;33(5):1027–30.

57. Mozo L, Gomez J, Escanlar E, et al. Diagnostic value of anti-deamidated gliadin peptide IgG antibodies for celiac disease in children and IgA-deficient patients. J Pediatr Gastroenterol Nutr 2012;55(1):50–5.

58. Frulio G, Polimeno A, Palmieri D, et al. Evaluating diagnostic accuracy of anti-tissue Transglutaminase IgA antibodies as first screening for Celiac Disease in very young children. Clin Chim Acta 2015;446:237–40.

59. Mubarak A, Gmelig-Meyling FH, Wolters VM, et al. Immunoglobulin G antibodies against deamidated-gliadin-peptides outperform anti-endomysium and tissue transglutaminase antibodies in children <2 years age. APMIS 2011;119(12):894–900.

60. Richter T, Bossuyt X, Vermeersch P, et al. Determination of IgG and IgA antibodies against native gliadin is not helpful for the diagnosis of coeliac disease in children up to 2 years old. J Pediatr Gastroenterol Nutr 2012;55(1):21–5.

61. Olen O, Gudjonsdottir AH, Browaldh L, et al. Antibodies against deamidated gliadin peptides and tissue transglutaminase for diagnosis of pediatric celiac disease. J Pediatr Gastroenterol Nutr 2012;55(6):695–700.

62. Buckley RH, Dees SC, O'Fallon WM. Serum immunoglobulins. I. Levels in normal children and in uncomplicated childhood allergy. Pediatrics 1968;41(3):600–11.

63. Villalta D, Alessio MG, Tampoia M, et al. Testing for IgG class antibodies in celiac disease patients with selective IgA deficiency. A comparison of the diagnostic accuracy of 9 IgG anti-tissue transglutaminase, 1 IgG anti-gliadin and 1 IgG anti-deaminated gliadin peptide antibody assays. Clin Chim Acta 2007;382(1–2):95–9.

64. Absah I, Rishi AR, Gebrail R, et al. Lack of utility of anti-tTG IgG to diagnose celiac disease when anti-tTG IgA is negative. J Pediatr Gastroenterol Nutr 2017;64(5):726–9.

65. Hill ID, Fasano A, Guandalini S, et al. NASPGHAN clinical report on the diagnosis and treatment of gluten-related disorders. J Pediatr Gastroenterol Nutr 2016;63(1):156–65.

66. Prasad K, Thapa B, Nain C, et al. The frequency of histologic lesion variability of the duodenal mucosa in children with celiac disease. World J Pediatr 2010;6(1):60–4.

67. Werkstetter KJ, Korponay-Szabo IR, Popp A, et al. Accuracy in diagnosis of celiac disease without biopsies in clinical practice. Gastroenterology 2017;153(4):924–35.

68. Gidrewicz D, Potter K, Trevenen CL, et al. Evaluation of the ESPGHAN Celiac Guidelines in a North American Pediatric Population. Am J Gastroenterol 2015; 110(5):760–7.

69. Elitsur Y, Sigman T, Watkins R, et al. Tissue transglutaminase levels are not sufficient to diagnose celiac disease in North American practices without intestinal biopsies. Dig Dis Sci 2017;62(1):175–9.

70. Paul SP, Harries SL, Basude D. Barriers to implementing the revised ESPGHAN guidelines for coeliac disease in children: a cross-sectional survey of coeliac screen reporting in laboratories in England. Arch Dis Child 2017;102(10):942–6.

71. Harper J, Holleran S, Ramakrishnan R, et al. Anemia in celiac disease is multifactorial in etiology. Am J Hematol 2007;82(11):996–1000.

72. Halfdanarson T, Litzow M, Murray J. Hematologic manifestations of celiac disease. Blood 2007;109(2):412–21.

73. Abu Daya H, Lebwohl B, Lewis S, et al. Celiac disease patients presenting with anemia have more severe disease than those presenting with diarrhea. Clin Gastroenterol Hepatol 2013;11(11):1472–7.

74. Grisolano S, Oxentenko A, Murray J, et al. The usefulness of routine small bowel biopsies In evaluation of iron deficiency anemia. J Clin Gastroenterol 2004;38(9): 756–60.

75. Leffler D, Green P, Fasano A. Extraintestinal manifestations of coeliac disease. Nat Rev Gastroenterol Hepatol 2015;12:561–71.

76. Di Sabatino A, Rosado M, Cazzola P, et al. Splenic hypofunction and spectrum of autoimmune and malignant complications in celiac disease. Clin Gastroenterol Hepatol 2006;4(2):179–86.

77. Simons M, Scott-Sheldon L, Risech-Neyman Y, et al. Celiac disease and increased risk of pneumococcal infection: a systematic review and meta-analysis. Am J Med 2018;131(1):83–9.

78. Daron C, Soubrier M, Mathieu S. Occurrence of rheumatic symptoms in celiac disease: a meta-analysis: comment on the article "Osteoarticular manifestations of celiac disease and non-celiac gluten hypersensitivity" by Dos Santos and Liote. Joint Bone Spine 2017;84(5):645–6.

79. Collin P, Reunala T, Rasmussen M, et al. High incidence and prevalence of adult coeliac disease. Augmented diagnostic approach. Scand J Gastroenterol 1997; 32(11):1129–33.

80. Jakes A, Bradley S, Donlevy L. Dermatitis herpetiformis. BMJ 2014;348:g2557.

81. Nieri M, Tofani E, Defraia E, et al. Enamel defects and aphthous stomatitis in celiac and healthy subjects: systematic review and meta-analysis of controlled studies. J Dent 2017;65:1–10.

82. Souto-Souza D, da Consolacao Soares M, Rezende V, et al. Association between developmental defects of enamel and celiac disease: a meta-analysis. Arch Oral Biol 2018;87:180–90.

83. Hadjivassiliou M, Grunewald R, Sharrack B, et al. Gluten ataxia in perspective: epidemiology, genetic susceptibility and clinical characteristics. Brain 2003; 126(3):685–91.

84. Cicarelli G, Della Rocca G, Amboni M, et al. Clinical and neurological abnormalities in adult celiac disease. Neurol Sci 2003;24(5):311–7.

85. Bashiri H, Afshari D, Babaei N, et al. Celiac disease and epilepsy: the effect of gluten-free diet on seizure control. Adv Clin Exp Med 2016;25(4):751–4.

86. Esteve M, Temiño R, Carrasco A, et al. Potential coeliac disease markers and autoimmunity in olmesartan induced enteropathy: a population-based study. Dig Liver Dis 2016;48(2):154–61.

87. Wijarnpreecha K, Jaruvongvanich V, Cheungpasitpron W, et al. Association between celiac disease and schizophrenia: a meta-analysis. Eur J Gastroenterol Hepatol 2018;30(4):442–6.
88. Dima A, Jurcut C, Manolache A, et al. Hemorrhagic events in adult celiac disease patients. Case report and review of the literature. J Gastrointest Liver Dis 2018; 27(1):93–9.
89. Castillo N, Vanga R, Theethira T, et al. Prevalence of abnormal liver function tests in celiac disease and the effect of a gluten-free diet in the US population. Am J Gastroenterol 2015;110(8):1216–22.
90. Marciano F, Savoia M, Vajro P. Celiac disease-related hepatic injury: insights into associated conditions and underlying pathomechanisms. Dig Liver Dis 2016; 48(2):112–9.
91. Volta U, De Franceschi L, Lari F, et al. Coeliac disease hidden by cryptogenic hypertransaminasaemia. Lancet 1998;352(9121):26–9.
92. Kumar S, Gress F, Green P, et al. Chronic pancreatitis is a common finding in celiac patients who undergo endoscopic ultrasound. J Clin Gastroenterol 2016. [Epub ahead of print].
93. Sadr-Azodi O, Sanders D, Murray J, et al. Patients with celiac disease have an increased risk for pancreatitis. Clin Gastroenterol Hepatol 2012;10(10):1136–42.
94. Singh V, Haupt M, Geller D, et al. Less common etiologies of exocrine pancreatic insufficiency. World J Gastroenterol 2017;23(39):7059–76.
95. Tersigni C, Castellani R, de Waure C, et al. Celiac disease and reproductive disorders: meta-analysis of epidemiologic associations and potential pathogenic mechanisms. Hum Reprod Update 2014;20(4):582–93.
96. Cakmak E, Karakus S, Demirpence O, et al. Ovarian reserve assessment in celiac patients of reproductive age. Med Sci Monit 2018;24:1152–7.

Biopsy Diagnosis of Celiac Disease

The Pathologist's Perspective in Light of Recent Advances

Stephen M. Lagana, MD[a],*, Govind Bhagat, MD[b]

KEYWORDS

- Pathology • Celiac disease • Histopathology • Enteropathy • Differential diagnosis
- Duodenum

KEY POINTS

- Celiac disease remains a clinicopathologic diagnosis.
- The differential diagnosis for mild duodenal injury and severe duodenal injury is distinct.
- Small intestinal biopsies should be evaluated in a systematic and reproducible manner.
- Small intestinal biopsies for celiac disease should be reported in a systematic, reproducible way.
- Good communication between gastroenterologists and pathologists is key to establishing accurate diagnoses.

INTRODUCTION

Celiac disease (CD), also known as gluten-sensitive enteropathy, or celiac sprue is a common immune-mediated disorder that occurs in genetically predisposed individuals following consumption of certain grains, including wheat, which is characterized by a protean clinical syndrome and small intestinal mucosal inflammation.[1,2] Histopathologic abnormalities of small intestinal mucosa (intraepithelial lymphocytosis, lymphoplasmacytic inflammation of the lamina propria, villus atrophy, and crypt hyperplasia), now considered characteristic for CD, were first described by Paulley in 1954[3] (**Box 1**, **Fig. 1**). Because these alterations vary in severity, semiquantitative grading schemes have been developed, starting in the 1990s, when Marsh[4]

Disclosure Statement: No financial conflicts/disclosures for either author.
[a] Columbia University, New York Presbyterian Hospital, 622 West 168th Street, VC14-209, New York, NY 10032, USA; [b] Columbia University, New York Presbyterian Hospital, 622 West 168th Street, VC14-228, New York, NY 10032, USA
* Corresponding author.
E-mail address: SML2179@cumc.columbia.edu

Gastroenterol Clin N Am 48 (2019) 39–51
https://doi.org/10.1016/j.gtc.2018.09.003
0889-8553/19/© 2018 Elsevier Inc. All rights reserved.

Box 1
Histologic findings in active celiac disease

Intraepithelial lymphocytosis

Lymphoplasmacytic inflammation of lamina propria

Villus atrophy

Crypt hyperplasia

Granulocytic infiltrates (neutrophils and eosinophils)

Increased crypt apoptotic activity

Reactive epithelial changes

---

categorized the histologic patterns of small intestinal mucosal injury. This scheme was subsequently modified by Oberhuber in 1999 and the modified Marsh-Oberhuber classification is currently used by many pathologists, although newer simplified schemes have been suggested that are preferred by some (**Table 1**).[5,6] In our experience, as a referral center for the diagnosis and management of CD, we have noted that many pathologists do not assign a formal grade to the mucosal abnormalities. The reasons cited for this include interobserver variability in scoring the severity of mucosal alterations among pathologists and a lack of correlation between the degree of villus atrophy and clinical symptoms.[7,8] We find value in using grading schemes for several reasons. First, this allows for semiquantitative assessment of healing after initiation of gluten-free diet (GFD). Second, it allows for a convenient shorthand that describes all pertinent biopsy histopathologic features, provided all parties know which scheme is being referenced.

Beyond the aforementioned "classical" histologic features of active CD (ACD), there are additional findings that are common, although often overlooked. The enterocytes (absorptive intestinal epithelial cells) commonly have a reactive appearance, with mucin depletion, intracytoplasmic vacuolization, and a cuboidal rather than the typical columnar cell shape (**Fig. 2**).[9,10] Neutrophilic inflammation is common in the lamina propria, occurring in most newly diagnosed cases of ACD. This phenomenon has been shown to correlate with the degree of villus atrophy.[10] Activated eosinophils are increased in ACD.[11] Crypt apoptosis is often a subtle histologic finding. It is well described in autoimmune enteropathy (AE), mycophenolate toxicity, and

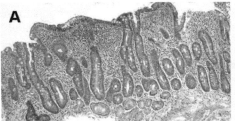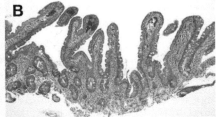

Fig. 1. Medium-power view of duodenal biopsy demonstrates the features of active celiac disease (*A*) and mucosal healing following approximately 18 months on a gluten-free diet (*B*). Note that in the active disease state the villi are completely atrophic and there is marked crypt hyperplasia. In the healed state, the architecture is normal and no inflammation is identified (hematoxylin and eosin, original magnification ×10).

Table 1 Comparison of the modified Marsh and Corazza-Villanacci grading schemes		
Histology	Marsh-Oberhuber Classification	Corazza-Villanacci Classification
Normal architecture, IEL	Type 1	Grade A
Normal villi, crypt hyperplasia + IEL	Type 2	
Partial VA + IEL	Type 3A	Grade B1
Subtotal VA + IEL	Type 3B	
Total VA	Type 3C	Grade B2
Hypoplastic lesion	Type 4	Deleted

Abbreviation: VA, villus atrophy.

graft-versus-host disease, but is also common in CD.[12] It is, however, important to note that these features although common in CD, are neither pathognomonic nor specific for it. Pathology outside of the small intestine may also be encountered in patients with CD, including microscopic colitis and lymphocytic or collagenous gastritis.[13,14] The ultimate diagnostic responsibility resides with the gastroenterologist who has to integrate the histopathologic findings with the clinical and endoscopic features, and laboratory results, including CD serology and potentially genetic testing.

A standardized approach to small intestinal biopsy procurement, interpretation, and reporting is beneficial to patient care. From the perspective of the gastrointestinal pathologist, it is our goal and responsibility to produce a report that it is accurate, clear, and complete while being free of extraneous (and potentially confusing) information. In our practice, we attempt to navigate these challenges by reviewing the histopathology and describing it without reviewing the history (to avoid bias). After the findings have been documented, the clinical notes/records are reviewed and an interpretive statement, including a differential diagnosis specific to the patient, is provided. When the clinical data are available, we believe these personalized reports provide more value than canned quick texts, which include every possible cause of the pattern of injury described.

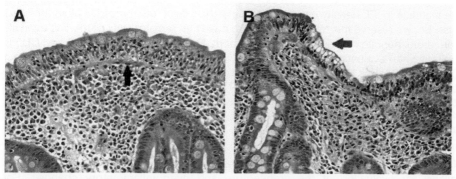

Fig. 2. (*A*) High-power view of a duodenal biopsy in the active disease state shows diffuse intraepithelial lymphocytosis. The IELs are seen above the *black arrow* (which indicates the subepithelial basement membrane). Beneath the *black arrow*, note that the lamina propria is packed with plasma cells. (*B*) Similar features with the additional finding of reactive epithelial changes (*red arrow*). Note the cytoplasmic vacuolization (hematoxylin and eosin, original magnification ×40).

APPROACH TO THE DUODENAL BIOPSY

There are three main phases in the "lifecycle" of a duodenal biopsy: (1) preanalytic, (2) analytical, and (3) postanalytic. Processes must be optimized and, ideally, standardized at each stage to ensure optimal results.

Preanalytic Phase

The most important preanalytic variable is biopsy sampling. This is for two reasons. First, like Crohn disease, mucosal alterations in CD can be patchy.[15] Second, small intestinal biopsies are not oriented before processing at most centers in the United States. It has been recommended that four to six biopsy pieces be obtained from both the second portion of the duodenum and duodenal bulb to ensure optimal sampling, especially when a diagnosis of CD is entertained.[15] The American College of Gastroenterology recommends acquiring biopsies from the postbulbar duodenum (four samples) and duodenal bulb (two samples), although it is well-known that many endoscopists do not procure the suggested number of biopsies, potentially leading to false-negative diagnoses.[16,17] One caveat to keep in mind is that the patient must be consuming gluten at the time of biopsy, because the negative predictive value of a normal-appearing biopsy is greatly reduced in the setting of a GFD.[16]

Biopsy of the duodenal bulb, previously disfavored because of the risk of artifacts (mainly from prominent Brunner glands) helps identify a small group of patients with CD (13%) who would be missed by postbulbar biopsies alone.[18] The quality of the biopsies may also be improved by taking one bite at a time to obtain the samples instead of multiple samples per pass. This strategy was shown to increase the yield of adequately oriented biopsies (66% vs 42%) in a prospective study.[19] Obtaining six levels from each small intestinal biopsy block (as opposed to the typical three levels for other types of gastrointestinal biopsies) is preferred for adequate evaluation. Hematoxylin and eosin staining of biopsies suffices for routine morphologic assessment. In our experience, immunohistochemistry (IHC) for T-cell antigens, specifically cluster of designation 3 (CD3), to highlight increased intraepithelial lymphocytes (IELs) is not useful in day-to-day practice.[20] Some investigators have suggested that CD3 IHC is "mandatory" in cases where IEL is suspected.[21] Some laboratories even perform CD3 IHC on all small intestinal biopsies "up-front," a practice that is contrary to evidence.[22] There are occasional cases, however, where CD3 IHC can accentuate a subtle increase in IEL density and may highlight their distribution mostly within the villus tips. So, we reserve this testing for the rare case that remains truly borderline even after careful hematoxylin and eosin assessment. Furthermore, IHC for CD3 and CD8 is helpful when evaluating for refractory CD. In such a setting, CD8 positivity by most (>50%) CD3$^+$ IELs is evidence against refractory CD type 2, a clonal lymphoproliferative disorder, or enteropathy-associated T-cell lymphoma, which are rare complications of CD (an in-depth review of these conditions has recently been published).[23]

Analytical Phase

The biopsy examination should begin with a careful and systematic low-power magnification ($\times 4$ objective) review of the slide evaluating all mucosal compartments. This allows for evaluation of the architecture and overt inflammatory changes. For adequate assessment, at least one biopsy piece should be "well-oriented," that is, four consecutive parallel crypt-villus units are visualized.[24] The interpreting pathologist must also know the range of normal morphologic variations of small intestinal mucosal architecture. In the duodenum, the villi should be three to five times taller than the crypts are deep.[25,26] If this ratio is not maintained, then there is villus atrophy and/or crypt hyperplasia. There are no guidelines to define an abnormal density of lamina propria lymphocytes and plasma cells. These are normal constituents of the intestinal lamina propria and their numbers increase in ACD and other inflammatory conditions. An experienced pathologist has a sense for what is normal and what is excessive. However, neutrophilic granulocytes are not considered a normal component of the small intestinal lamina propria.[27] The low-power evaluation should be completed by reviewing the space between the villi (if present) for parasites. *Giardia* organisms are often readily appreciated on low-magnification, but can be missed if the biopsy is not reviewed in a systematic manner.

After the completion of the low-power review, all biopsies should be subjected to high magnification evaluation. The purpose of this is to examine features that may not be readily appreciated at low power including IEL density, presence of goblet and Paneth cells, presence of gastric metaplasia and heterotopia, presence of subepithelial fibrosis, presence and qualitative assessment of granulocytes, presence and qualitative assessment of plasma cells, and presence of pathogens. Although there is some disagreement in the literature about the normal number of IELs in the duodenum, most experts accept up to 25 per 100 enterocytes.[28] An increase greater than this level constitutes IEL. The distribution of the IELs is also relevant. Normal duodenal mucosa has a "decrescendo" pattern of IELs, with a greater density present at the basal portion of the of villi.[29] Because of this, it has been shown that increased IELs at the tips of villi (defined as a mean of 12 IELs per 20 enterocytes in five villus tips) correlate with CD, whereas IEL increases along the lateral edges of villi are less specific.[29] This altered pattern may also be useful in identifying patients with potential CD (seropositivity without symptoms or villus atrophy).[30] The normal and pathologic IEL distribution patterns and an increase in IELs cannot be adequately assessed in unoriented biopsies or when the villi are detached or completely atrophic.

Once the low- and high-power examination is complete, the observations should be organized in a consistent fashion. Definitive statements should be made whenever possible (eg, "Duodenal mucosa, within normal limits," or "Duodenal mucosa with giardiasis"). It is not uncommon to identify inflammatory changes, which suggest a disease, but are not independently diagnostic. In such settings, a differential diagnosis should be included in the report. If the pathologist has access to the medical records, and/or to the gastroenterologist, the differential should be tailored to the patient's circumstances.

DIFFERENTIAL DIAGNOSIS

It is helpful to think of the differential diagnosis of CD in relation to the Marsh-Oberhuber pattern. Put another way, when a pathologist is considering a Marsh-Oberhuber type 1 pattern (normal architecture and increased IELs), the differential is different from when a Marsh-Oberhuber type 3C pattern (flat mucosa) is encountered. The common differential diagnoses are summarized in **Table 2**.

Preserved Architecture with Intraepithelial Lymphocytosis

The differential diagnosis of Marsh-Oberhuber type 1 (or Corazza A) pattern is broad. This pattern has been detected with increasing frequency in recent years. As the rate of detection of increased IELs, the positive predictive value of this pattern with respect to CD has decreased.[31] Many cases are idiopathic; however, other etiologies include partially treated CD, tropical sprue, *Helicobacter pylori* infection (of the stomach), medication/drug effect (proton pump inhibitors, selective serotonin reuptake inhibitors, nonsteroidal anti-inflammatory drugs, and others), small intestinal

Table 2	
Histologic differential diagnosis based on pattern	
Normal Villus Architecture and Increased IELs	**Villus Atrophy With/Without Increased IELs**
Celiac disease	Celiac disease, and complicated celiac
Helicobacter pylori–associated	disease (eg, refractory sprue,
gastroduodenitis	collagenous sprue)
Drugs: NSAIDs, selective serotonin reuptake	Angiotensin receptor blocker–associated
inhibitors, proton pump inhibitor	enteropathy
Tropical sprue	Drugs: mycophenolate mofetil, colchicine
Infections, such as viral enteritis, *Giardia*,	Immune dysregulation: autoimmune
Cryptosporidium	enteropathy
Immune conditions: rheumatoid arthritis,	Immunodeficiency: common variable
Hashimoto thyroiditis, SLE, autoimmune	immune deficiency
enteropathy	Graft-versus-host disease
Immunodeficiency: common variable immune	Inflammatory bowel disease
deficiency	Chemoradiation therapy
Graft-versus-host disease	Nutritional deficiency
Inflammatory bowel disease	Eosinophilic enteritis
Small intestinal bacterial overgrowth	Lymphoma
Irritable bowel syndrome	

Abbreviations: NSAID, nonsteroidal anti-inflammatory drug; SLE, systemic lupus erythematosus.

bacterial overgrowth, infections (viral gastroenteritis), morbid obesity, autoimmune disorders, inflammatory bowel disease, and others.[31–38] Because some of the etiologic factors are common (eg, medication use) and the patient might have more than one pathologic condition, it is challenging to determine the instigating/causative agents. Detailed clinical information and laboratory studies (including genetic testing) may be needed to exclude CD in such instances. In a patient with known history of CD, it is reasonable to attribute this finding to minimal gluten exposure. In the setting of newly diagnosed CD, this pattern is uncommon.[10] Studies suggest that 5% to 10% of patients without a known history of CD whose biopsies exhibit the Marsh-Oberhuber type 1 pattern will ultimately be determined to have CD.[10,39] However, in one study, approximately 16% of children with abdominal pain, but without CD, *H pylori* gastritis, or other identifiable gastrointestinal disease, had more than 25 IELs per 100 enterocytes.[40] Thus, when a clinician receives a pathology report describing a Marsh-Oberhuber type 1 pattern, it is prudent to perform further studies to exclude CD, but one should recognize that this finding is common, nonspecific, and often idiopathic.

Villus Atrophy

The presence of villus atrophy is a more concerning finding, which should not be accepted as "idiopathic" without significant consideration and potentially referral to a specialized center. The differential of villus atrophy and increased IELs includes CD; medication-related enteropathy, particularly the recently described olmesartan-associated enteropathy (OAE) (occasionally also associated with other angiotensin receptor blockers [ARBs]), mycophenolate-containing compounds, and colchicine among others; collagenous sprue; common variable immunodeficiency; AE; lymphoma, inflammatory bowel disease; and certain infections.[41]

Of these entities, the one that has garnered the most attention recently is OAE. Rubio-Tapia and colleagues[42] reported a series of 22 patients who presented with severe diarrhea and profound weight loss following exposure to olmesartan. Biopsies of the small intestine showed severe villus atrophy and inflammation. Fifteen had total villus atrophy and 14 had increased IELs. Serologic testing for CD was universally negative and GFD did not resolve symptoms or mucosal abnormalities. Seven patients had collagenous sprue. Of 14 patients who also had gastric biopsies, five (36%) exhibited lymphocytic gastritis and two (14%) displayed features of collagenous gastritis. Colon biopsies of 5 of the 13 patients (38%) showed microscopic colitis (two lymphocytic, three collagenous). Clinical symptoms resolved quickly following cessation of the medications in all cases, and the histologic changes disappeared in most.[42] Several additional case reports, series, and reviews have confirmed these findings and implicated other ARBs.[41,43–59] The US Food and Drug Administration approved a label change for olmesartan in 2013 to acknowledge the risk of enteropathy.[60]

As is deduced from the preceding description of the histopathology of OAE, it is difficult (sometimes impossible) to distinguish OAE from ACD based on morphologic features alone. In a subset of OAE cases, there are histologic clues that should allow the attentive pathologist to suggest the diagnosis. The first is the density of IELs. Studies have shown that some ARB-enteropathy cases do not display significant increased IELs, a feature that is essentially universal in ACD.[42,59] Second, OAE cases commonly demonstrate increased subepithelial collagen (collagenous sprue-like features), which is a rare finding in CD (**Fig. 3**).[41,42,61] Ultimately, seronegativity and medication exposure are the most meaningful data points in distinguishing between CD and ARB-enteropathy and clinical and histopathologic response to a change of medication class supports medication exposure as the inciting insult. As such, OAE is a good example of a situation in which knowing the clinical history allows the pathologist to make a more meaningful statement regarding the cause and the appropriate diagnosis.

Common variable immunodeficiency is an immunodeficiency disorder characterized by the failure of B cell maturation into plasma cells, causing decreased serum immunoglobulin levels. Patients may present with diarrhea and malabsorption and are prone to infections (giardiasis and bacterial overgrowth).[62,63] Duodenal biopsies can demonstrate a variety of changes, including increased IELs and variable degrees of villus atrophy.[64] Common variable immunodeficiency typically displays an absence or severe decrease in the number of lamina propria plasma cells. This is in contrast to

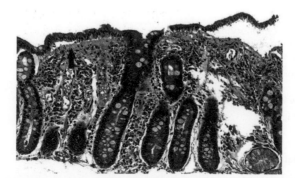

Fig. 3. This patient presented with intractable diarrhea and profound weight loss. Duodenal biopsy showed total villus atrophy, as is seen in celiac disease. Notably, the subepithelial collagen layer was thickened (*arrow*), and the epithelium seemed to slough off. This diagnostic clue coupled with the lack of intraepithelial lymphocytosis suggested a diagnosis of olmesartan-associated enteropathy. Discussion at an interdisciplinary conference confirmed medication exposure with negative celiac serology, and the patient responded dramatically to a medication change (hematoxylin and eosin, original magnification ×40).

Box 2
Template used to describe findings in small intestinal biopsies performed for evaluatlon of celiac disease

I. Clinical Information
   None provided
   Rule out celiac disease
   Previous diagnosis of celiac disease
   Refractory celiac disease
   Other (specify): _____

II. Type of Mucosa
   Duodenal
   Jejunal

III. Number of Biopsy Pieces
   _____

IV. Adequacy of Specimen Orientation (at least four consecutive well-oriented crypt-villus units)
   Yes
   No

V. Villus Length
   Normal
   Abnormal
   Cannot be determined

VI. Crypt Length
   Normal
   Elongated
   Shortened

VII. Crypt-to-Villus Ratio
   Normal (1:3–1:5)
   Abnormal (specify):_____

VIII. Villus Atrophy
   None
   Total
   Subtotal
   Partial
   Diffuse
   Patchy

IX. Intraepithelial Lymphocytes
   Normal (up to 30 per 100 epithelial nuclei)
   Increased, specify: mild, moderate, severe, focal, diffuse

X. Lamina Propria Inflammatory Cells
   Normal
   Increased, specify: plasma cells, eosinophils, lymphocytes, neutrophils

XI. Gastric Metaplasia
   Present
   Absent

XII. Subepithelial Collagen
   Normal
   Increased

XIII. Diagnosis
   Small intestinal mucosa, histologically unremarkable
   Focal chronic inflammation with or without focal intraepithelial lymphocytes, nonspecific
   Diffuse intraepithelial lymphocytosis, normal villi, consistent with celiac disease (Marsh type 1)

Diffuse intraepithelial lymphocytosis and crypt hyperplasia, consistent with celiac disease (Marsh type 2)

Partial villus atrophy, crypt hyperplasia and intraepithelial lymphocytosis, consistent with celiac disease (Marsh type 3a)

Subtotal villus atrophy, crypt hyperplasia and intraepithelial lymphocytosis, consistent with celiac disease (Marsh type 3b)

Total villus atrophy, crypt hyperplasia and intraepithelial lymphocytosis, consistent with celiac disease (Marsh type 3c)

Villus atrophy, crypt hypoplasia and intraepithelial lymphocytosis, consistent with celiac disease (Marsh type 4)

CD, where the plasma cells are increased. At times, the increase of lamina propria lymphocytes may be significant, making it difficult to discern the lack of plasma cells.

The term "autoimmune enteropathy" refers to a group of rare autoimmune conditions which primarily afflict infants, but can also rarely present in adults. In young males, an X-linked severe form of the disorder is associated with immune dysregulation and polyendocrinopathy caused by a germline mutation in the FOXP3 gene located on the X chromosome.[65] Patients with this disease may present with failure to thrive, secretory diarrhea, weight loss, and malabsorption, requiring total parental nutrition. AE commonly affects the proximal small bowel, with involvement of the stomach, distal small bowel, and colon described in some cases. Duodenal biopsies show variable villus atrophy and crypt hyperplasia, often with a diminished number of Paneth and goblet cells. A dense lymphoplasmacytic infiltrate in the lamina propria is common and neutrophils with crypt abscesses are seen in severe cases.[66–68] Although an increase in IELs may be seen, this is more prominent in the crypts. This feature may help distinguish AE from CD, which usually demonstrates marked increase in surface IELs.[67] Crypt apoptosis is often prominent in AE, although again, this finding is not specific because it is identified in other disorders and CD.[12] Laboratory tests may demonstrate the presence of antienterocyte antibodies and some patients may also have anti–goblet cell, anti–parietal cell, and anti–smooth muscle antibodies. Antigliadin and antireticulin antibodies have also been described in AE.[68] We have encountered a case of OAE where the ileal biopsy showed near total loss of goblet and Paneth cells, raising suspicion for AE. However, these cells were readily identified on a subsequent biopsy after olmesartan was discontinued.[45] There is considerable morphologic overlap in these entities, highlighting the importance of attention to detail and clinical correlation.

POSTANALYTIC PHASE

Postanalytic variables in the context of duodenal biopsies mainly concern reporting terminology. Many centers use "quick texts" to describe gastrointestinal biopsy findings; however, important information is often missed as a consequence.[7] To ensure that all relevant data are conveyed in pathology reports, we use a worksheet for biopsies, which come with a request to assess for CD or to evaluate the cause of persistent symptoms or response to therapy (Box 2). The idea is to use a scheme similar to tumor staging checklists, and analogous to the staging forms. Our worksheet was developed as a collaboration between clinicians and pathologists.

SUMMARY

We have described an approach to the duodenal biopsy and discussed considerations related to the differential diagnosis and optimal reporting of CD. Although a clinicopathologic diagnosis of CD may be straightforward in many instances, there are also many opportunities for confusion and error. Good communication between gastroenterologist and pathologist is vital for accurate diagnosis. This is achieved via access to comprehensive notes or reports in the electronic medical record, communication by e-mails or telephone calls, and ideally, by participating in interdisciplinary conferences.

REFERENCES

1. Dicke WK, Weijers HA, Van De Kamer JH. Coeliac disease. II. The presence in wheat of a factor having a deleterious effect in cases of coeliac disease. Acta Paediatr 1953;42(1):34–42.
2. Abadie V, Sollid LM, Barreiro LB, et al. Integration of genetic and immunological insights into a model of celiac disease pathogenesis. Annu Rev Immunol 2011; 29:493–525.
3. Paulley JW. Observation on the aetiology of idiopathic steatorrhoea; jejunal and lymph-node biopsies. Br Med J 1954;2(4900):1318–21.
4. Marsh MN. Gluten, major histocompatibility complex, and the small intestine. A molecular and immunobiologic approach to the spectrum of gluten sensitivity ('celiac sprue'). Gastroenterology 1992;102(1):330–54.
5. Oberhuber G, Granditsch G, Vogelsang H. The histopathology of coeliac disease: time for a standardized report scheme for pathologists. Eur J Gastroenterol Hepatol 1999;11(10):1185–94.
6. Corazza GR, Villanacci V, Zambelli C, et al. Comparison of the interobserver reproducibility with different histologic criteria used in celiac disease. Clin Gastroenterol Hepatol 2007;5(7):838–43.
7. Arguelles-Grande C, Tennyson CA, Lewis SK, et al. Variability in small bowel histopathology reporting between different pathology practice settings: impact on the diagnosis of coeliac disease. J Clin Pathol 2012;65(3):242–7.
8. Brar P, Kwon GY, Egbuna II, et al. Lack of correlation of degree of villus atrophy with severity of clinical presentation of coeliac disease. Dig Liver Dis 2007;39(1): 26–9 [discussion: 30–2].
9. Bao F, Green PH, Bhagat G. An update on celiac disease histopathology and the road ahead. Arch Pathol Lab Med 2012;136(7):735–45.
10. Brown IS, Smith J, Rosty C. Gastrointestinal pathology in celiac disease: a case series of 150 consecutive newly diagnosed patients. Am J Clin Pathol 2012; 138(1):42–9.
11. Colombel JF, Torpier G, Janin A, et al. Activated eosinophils in adult coeliac disease: evidence for a local release of major basic protein. Gut 1992;33(9):1190–4.
12. Shalimar DM, Das P, Sreenivas V, et al. Mechanism of villus atrophy in celiac disease: role of apoptosis and epithelial regeneration. Arch Pathol Lab Med 2013; 137(9):1262–9.
13. Green PH, Yang J, Cheng J, et al. An association between microscopic colitis and celiac disease. Clin Gastroenterol Hepatol 2009;7(11):1210–6.
14. Carmack SW, Lash RH, Gulizia JM, et al. Lymphocytic disorders of the gastrointestinal tract: a review for the practicing pathologist. Adv Anat Pathol 2009;16(5): 290–306.
15. Hopper AD, Cross SS, Sanders DS. Patchy villus atrophy in adult patients with suspected gluten-sensitive enteropathy: is a multiple duodenal biopsy strategy appropriate? Endoscopy 2008;40(3):219–24.

16. Rubio-Tapia A, Hill ID, Kelly CP, et al. ACG clinical guidelines: diagnosis and management of celiac disease. Am J Gastroenterol 2013;108(5):656–76 [quiz: 677].
17. Lebwohl B, Kapel RC, Neugut AI, et al. Adherence to biopsy guidelines increases celiac disease diagnosis. Gastrointest Endosc 2011;74(1):103–9.
18. Gonzalez S, Gupta A, Cheng J, et al. Prospective study of the role of duodenal bulb biopsies in the diagnosis of celiac disease. Gastrointest Endosc 2010; 72(4):758–65.
19. Latorre M, Lagana SM, Freedberg DE, et al. Endoscopic biopsy technique in the diagnosis of celiac disease: one bite or two? Gastrointest Endosc 2015;81(5): 1228–33.
20. Mino M, Lauwers GY. Role of lymphocytic immunophenotyping in the diagnosis of gluten-sensitive enteropathy with preserved villus architecture. Am J Surg Pathol 2003;27(9):1237–42.
21. Volta U, Villanacci V. Celiac disease: diagnostic criteria in progress. Cell Mol Immunol 2011;8(2):96–102.
22. Hudacko R, Kathy Zhou X, Yantiss RK. Immunohistochemical stains for CD3 and CD8 do not improve detection of gluten-sensitive enteropathy in duodenal biopsies. Mod Pathol 2013;26(9):1241–5.
23. Chander U, Leeman-Neill RJ, Bhagat G. Pathogenesis of enteropathy-associated T cell lymphoma. Curr Hematol Malig Rep 2018;13(4):308–17.
24. Perera DR, Weinstein WM, Rubin CE. Symposium on pathology of the gastrointestinal tract-part II. Small intestinal biopsy. Hum Pathol 1975;6(2):157–217.
25. Serra S, Jani PA. An approach to duodenal biopsies. J Clin Pathol 2006;59: 1133–50.
26. Dickson BC, Streutker CJ, Chetty R. Coeliac disease: an update for pathologists. J Clin Pathol 2006;59(10):1008–16.
27. Villanacci V, Ceppa P, Tavani E, et al. Coeliac disease: the histology report. Dig Liver Dis 2011;43(Suppl 4):S385–95.
28. Hayat M, Cairns A, Dixon MF, et al. Quantitation of intraepithelial lymphocytes in human duodenum: what is normal? J Clin Pathol 2002;55(5):393–4.
29. Goldstein NS, Underhill J. Morphologic features suggestive of gluten sensitivity in architecturally normal duodenal biopsy specimens. Am J Clin Pathol 2001;116(1): 63–71.
30. Biagi F, Luinetti O, Campanella J, et al. Intraepithelial lymphocytes in the villus tip: do they indicate potential coeliac disease? J Clin Pathol 2004;57(8):835–9.
31. Shmidt E, Smyrk TC, Boswell CL, et al. Increasing duodenal intraepithelial lymphocytosis found at upper endoscopy: time trends and associations. Gastrointest Endosc 2014;80(1):105–11.
32. Memeo L, Jhang J, Hibshoosh H, et al. Duodenal intraepithelial lymphocytosis with normal villus architecture: common occurrence in H. pylori gastritis. Mod Pathol 2005;18(8):1134–44.
33. Harpaz N, Levi GS, Yurovitsky A, et al. Intraepithelial lymphocytosis in architecturally normal small intestinal mucosa: association with morbid obesity. Arch Pathol Lab Med 2007;131(3):344 [author reply: 344].
34. Brown IS, Bettington A, Bettington M, et al. Tropical sprue: revisiting an underrecognized disease. Am J Surg Pathol 2014;38(5):666–72.
35. Masia R, Peyton S, Lauwers GY, et al. Gastrointestinal biopsy findings of autoimmune enteropathy: a review of 25 cases. Am J Surg Pathol 2014;38(10): 1319–29.

36. Patterson ER, Shmidt E, Oxentenko AS, et al. Normal villus architecture with increased intraepithelial lymphocytes: a duodenal manifestation of Crohn disease. Am J Clin Pathol 2015;143(3):445–50.
37. Lauwers GY, Fasano A, Brown IS. Duodenal lymphocytosis with no or minimal enteropathy: much ado about nothing? Mod Pathol 2015;28(Suppl 1):S22–9.
38. Aziz I, Evans KE, Hopper AD, et al. A prospective study into the aetiology of lymphocytic duodenosis. Aliment Pharmacol Ther 2010;32(11–12):1392–7.
39. Kakar S, Nehra V, Murray JA, et al. Significance of intraepithelial lymphocytosis in small bowel biopsy samples with normal mucosal architecture. Am J Gastroenterol 2003;98(9):2027–33.
40. Guz-Mark A, Zevit N, Morgenstern S, et al. Duodenal intraepithelial lymphocytosis is common in children without coeliac disease, and is not meaningfully influenced by Helicobacter pylori infection. Aliment Pharmacol Ther 2014;39(11):1314–20.
41. DeGaetani M, Tennyson CA, Lebwohl B, et al. villus atrophy and negative celiac serology: a diagnostic and therapeutic dilemma. Am J Gastroenterol 2013; 108(5):647–53.
42. Rubio-Tapia A, Herman ML, Ludvigsson JF, et al. Severe spruelike enteropathy associated with olmesartan. Mayo Clin Proc 2012;87(8):732–8.
43. Malfertheiner P, Ripellino C, Cataldo N. Severe intestinal malabsorption associated with ACE inhibitor or angiotensin receptor blocker treatment. An observational cohort study in Germany and Italy. Pharmacoepidemiol Drug Saf 2018; 27(6):581–6.
44. Abdelghany M, Gonzalez L 3rd, Slater J, et al. Olmesartan associated sprue-like enteropathy and colon perforation. Case Rep Gastrointest Med 2014;2014: 494098.
45. Burbure N, Lebwohl B, Arguelles-Grande C, et al. Olmesartan-associated sprue-like enteropathy: a systematic review with emphasis on histopathology. Hum Pathol 2016;50:127–34.
46. de Fonseka A, Tuskey A, Moskaluk C. A case of olmesartan induced enteropathy. Inflamm Bowel Dis 2012;18(S17).
47. Dreifuss SE, Tomizawa Y, Farber NJ, et al. Spruelike enteropathy associated with olmesartan: an unusual case of severe diarrhea. Case Rep Gastrointest Med 2013;2013:618071.
48. Fiorucci G, Puxeddu E, Colella R, et al. Severe spruelike enteropathy due to olmesartan. Rev Esp Enferm Dig 2014;106(2):142–4.
49. Freeman HJ. Olmesartan enteropathy. IJCD 2016;4(1):24–6.
50. Herman M, Rubio-Tapia A, Wu TT, et al. ACG Case Rep J 2015;2(2):92–4.
51. Khan AS, Peter S, Wilcox CM. Olmesartan-induced enteropathy resembling celiac disease. Endoscopy 2014;46(Suppl 1 UCTN):E97–8.
52. Marthey L, Cadiot G, Seksik P, et al. Olmesartan-associated enteropathy: results of a national survey. Aliment Pharmacol Ther 2014;40(9):1103–9.
53. Nielsen JA, Steephen A, Lewin M. Angiotensin-II inhibitor (olmesartan)-induced collagenous sprue with resolution following discontinuation of drug. World J Gastroenterol 2013;19(40):6928–30.
54. Scialom S, Malamut G, Meresse B, et al. Gastrointestinal disorder associated with olmesartan mimics autoimmune enteropathy. PLoS One 2015;10(6):e0125024.
55. Stanich PP, Yearsley M, Meyer MM. Olmesartan-associated sprue-like enteropathy. J Clin Gastroenterol 2013;47(10):894–5.
56. Talbot GH. Small bowel histopathologic findings suggestive of celiac disease in an asymptomatic patient receiving olmesartan. Mayo Clin Proc 2012;87(12): 1231–2 [author reply: 1232].

57. Theophile H, David XR, Miremont-Salame G, et al. Five cases of sprue-like enteropathy in patients treated by olmesartan. Dig Liver Dis 2014;46(5):465–9.
58. Tran TH, Li H. Olmesartan and drug-induced enteropathy. P T 2014;39(1):47–50.
59. Ianiro G, Bibbo S, Montalto M, et al. Systematic review: sprue-like enteropathy associated with olmesartan. Aliment Pharmacol Ther 2014;40(1):16–23.
60. FDA. U.S. Food and Drug Administration. FDA Drug Safety Communication: FDA approves label changes to include intestinal problems (sprue-like enteropathy) linked to blood pressure medicine olmesartan medoxomil. 2013. Available at: http://www.fda.gov/drugs/drugsafety/ucm359477.htm. Accessed June 19, 2014.
61. Vakiani E, Arguelles-Grande C, Mansukhani MM, et al. Collagenous sprue is not always associated with dismal outcomes: a clinicopathological study of 19 patients. Mod Pathol 2010;23(1):12–26.
62. Ament ME, Ochs HD, Davis SD. Structure and function of the gastrointestinal tract in primary immunodeficiency syndromes. A study of 39 patients. Medicine 1973; 52(3):227–48.
63. Washington K, Stenzel TT, Buckley RH, et al. Gastrointestinal pathology in patients with common variable immunodeficiency and X-linked agammaglobulinemia. Am J Surg Pathol 1996;20(10):1240–52.
64. Malamut G, Verkarre V, Suarez F, et al. The enteropathy associated with common variable immunodeficiency: the delineated frontiers with celiac disease. Am J Gastroenterol 2010;105(10):2262–75.
65. Le Bras S, Geha RS. IPEX and the role of Foxp3 in the development and function of human Tregs. J Clin Invest 2006;116(6):1473–5.
66. Montalto M, D'Onofrio F, Santoro L, et al. Autoimmune enteropathy in children and adults. Scand J Gastroenterol 2009;44(9):1029–36.
67. Russo PA, Brochu P, Seidman EG, et al. Autoimmune enteropathy. Pediatr Dev Pathol 1999;2(1):65–71.
68. Corazza GR, Biagi F, Volta U, et al. Autoimmune enteropathy and villus atrophy in adults. Lancet 1997;350(9071):106–9.

Nutritional Considerations of the Gluten-Free Diet

Melinda Dennis, MS, RDN, LD[a], Anne R. Lee, EdD, RDN, LD[b],*,
Tara McCarthy, MS, RDN[c]

KEYWORDS

- Gluten-free diet • Nutrient deficiencies • Nonresponsive celiac disease
- Quality of life • Nutrition therapy • Obesity

KEY POINTS

- A registered dietitian is uniquely qualified to educate on the gluten-free diet (GFD) and to assess and support nutritional status at diagnosis and long term.
- Because of the nutritional deficiencies inherent in the GFD, it should only be used in the treatment of gluten-related disorders.
- Celiac disease and the GFD have been associated with decreased quality of life; registered dietitian nutritionists can assess and support at diagnosis and long term.
- Causes of nonresponsive celiac disease include gluten exposure, small intestinal bacterial overgrowth, irritable bowel syndrome, lactose intolerance, microscopic colitis, food allergies, eating disorders, disaccharide deficiency, and refractory celiac disease.

INTRODUCTION

Celiac disease (CD) is a genetically mediated autoimmune disease in which gluten causes intestinal inflammation or damage. The prevalence of CD in the United States is 1:141, similar to several European countries.[1] Historically, CD has been underdiagnosed; however, the rate of diagnosis is increasing.[2] There is a disproportionate increase in growth of the gluten-free (GF) market compared with the increase in the prevalence of CD, indicating the growing use of the GF diet (GFD) in the absence of a diagnosis.[3] A 2012 study of 579 children and adolescents without CD found that 7.4% were following the GFD for irritability, family history of CD, bowel movement changes, diarrhea, and autism.[4] In contrast with the trend, for individuals with CD,

Disclosure: See last page of article.
[a] Celiac Center, Beth Israel Deaconess Medical Center, 330 Brookline Avenue, Dana 603, Boston, MA 02215, USA; [b] Celiac Disease Center at Columbia University Medical Center, Harkness Pavilion, 180 Fort Washington Avenue, 9th Floor, Suite 936, New York, NY 10032, USA; [c] Division of Gastroenterology, Hepatology and Nutrition, Celiac Center, Boston Children's Hospital, 330 Longwood Avenue, Boston, MA 02215, USA
* Corresponding author.
E-mail address: arl2004@cumc.columbia.edu

there are nutritional concerns of the GFD, including nutritional deficiencies, quality of life (QOL), and weight gain. Patients receive information from many different sources and, with the increase in popularity of the GFD, it is imperative that patients with CD are managed by a team approach, including a registered dietitian nutritionist (RDN) skilled in CD.[5]

ROLE OF THE REGISTERED DIETITIAN NUTRITIONIST

Consultation with an RDN skilled in CD is one of the 6 main principles set forth by the US National Institutes of Health (NIH) for CD[5] and includes a full assessment of the patient's medical and social history; identification of potential nutrient deficiencies or excesses with a thorough diet assessment[6,7]; diet education; and development of an individualized, balanced nutrition treatment plan for symptoms and comorbidities. Ongoing follow-up is essential to assess knowledge level, diet compliance, and nutritional status, and to provide clinical updates and guidance on navigating social and emotional aspects of the GF lifestyle.[7]

GLUTEN-FREE DIET BASICS

Gluten is a protein found in wheat, barley, and rye that provides structure and elasticity. Gluten-containing foods typically include breads, pasta, cereals, baked goods, and beverages. Corn, rice, and potato have been the traditional substitutes for a GFD. Removing gluten-containing grains can diminish the nutrient content of the GFD, specifically minerals, B vitamins, and fiber (**Table 1**). A GFD requires the elimination of all gluten; however, it is imperative to focus on the individual's total intake, not just the gluten.

Emphasizing the naturally GF foods such as fruits, vegetables, plant and animal sources of protein, dairy, fats, and oils provides a sound nutritional base. The addition of the alternative naturally GF whole grains such as amaranth and quinoa provides the fiber, B vitamins, and minerals missing when gluten is removed. A GFD prescription should include standard nutritional guidance emphasizing the use of fresh fruits, vegetables, whole grains, and less processed foods.[8] In addition, the standard distribution of calories as 50% to 60% from carbohydrate, focusing on complex carbohydrates and whole grains; 30% to 35% from fats, emphasizing foods rich in omega 3 and 6; and 10% to 15% of calories from protein, with a variety of both animal and plant sources, ensures a balanced nutrient intake.

LABEL READING

In the United States, the Food Allergen Labeling and Consumer Protection Act (FALCPA) requires food labels to identify the 8 major food allergens, including wheat.[9] The law clearly identifies wheat, and its derivatives, but does not include barley or rye or their derivatives (see **Table 1**). The US Food and Drug Administration (FDA) has defined GF as a food that is either inherently GF or has been processed to remove gluten to less than 20 parts per million (ppm), including ingredients and cross-contact.[10] In FDA-regulated products, the presence of wheat must be declared on the label. However, "wheat free" on a label does not mean GF. Educating patients to carefully read labels for any potential gluten is crucial. Manufacturers can change ingredients without notification. The US Department of Agriculture (USDA), which may or may not comply with the voluntary FALCPA guidelines, regulates meat products, poultry products, egg products, and mixed food products that generally contain a percentage of raw or cooked meat or chicken products.[11]

Table 1
General foods to include and avoid on a healthy, balanced, and safe gluten-free diet

Foods to Include	Foods to Avoid
Grains and grain-based products[a]	Wheat
Provide fiber, zinc, iron, B complex vitamins	Staple in breads, cereals, pasta, cakes, cookies, and many snacks
Amaranth	Soy sauce unless labeled GF
Arrowroot	Licorice (if made with wheat)
Buckwheat	Wheat flour can be used in gravies,
Corn	sauces, soups, and thickening agents
Millet	Barley
Oats (see oats section)	Barley (flakes, flour, pearl)
Quinoa	Malt (flavoring, vinegar, extract, syrup)
Rice: all varieties	Brown rice syrup (if made with malt)
Sorghum	Yeast extract/autolyzed yeast extract
Tapioca	(if made with barley)
Teff	Beer, lager, ale (unless labeled GF)
Flours from nontraditional sources	Brewer's yeast
Bean flour: chickpea, lentil, soy	Rye
Nut flour: almond, chestnut, coconut	Rye flour, bread, and flavoring (not
Seed flour: flax meal	typically a flavor enhancer or binder)
	Oats
	Oats not labeled GF (see text)
Dairy	Yogurt with cookie crumb or granola
Provides calcium, vitamin D, phosphorus, and protein	topping if not labeled GF
Animal protein	Avoid marinated, breaded, or coated
Provides iron, niacin, zinc, B$_{12}$, riboflavin, vitamin A	Caution:
	• Deli meat
	• Sausages, hot dogs
	• Prepared meats
Vegetable protein	Dried beans should be thoroughly
Provides fiber and essential fatty acids	sorted, rinsed, and drained
Beans and legumes: folic acid	Choose plain nuts and seeds
Nuts/nut butters: magnesium, calcium, iron	
Seeds/seed butters: iron, copper, selenium, zinc	
Fruits and vegetables	Vegetables in sauces
Provides vitamin C, folic acid, vitamin A	
A variety of deep red, purple, and dark green fruits and vegetables should be used, including starchy vegetables such as sweet potatoes and corn	
Fats and oil	—
Provide vitamin E	
Sugar and sweets	Licorice (made with wheat flour)
	Candies with crispy or cookie ingredients
Sauces	Soy sauce not labeled GF

This list is not comprehensive and not a substitute for RDN consultation.
  [a] All grains, flours, starches, and grain-based products should be labeled GF. Plain rice is the exception.

Many traditional foods used for holidays, religious ceremonies, and cultural celebrations may contain gluten. GF and low-gluten communion wafers and unleavened, GF, oat-based matzo are available in the marketplace. Resources for patients regarding CD and the GF diet can be found in **Table 2**.

LABELING NONFOOD ITEMS

Nonfood items do not follow the same labeling laws and may contain gluten. Gluten is not absorbed through intact skin.[12] Body care products applied to the skin and hair (body lotion, sunscreen, shaving cream, deodorant, makeup, perfume, shampoo, and conditioner) do not seem to be a concern, particularly if hands are washed after

Table 2 Celiac disease resources	
Resource	**URL**
Academy of Nutrition and Dietetics: Evidence Analysis Library	https://www.eatrightpro.org/research/applied-practice/evidence-analysis-library
Beyond Celiac	https://www.beyondceliac.org
Celiac Disease Foundation	https://www.celiac.org
Feeding America	https://www.feedingamerica.org/find-your-local-foodbank Find your local Food Bank and then ask about GF options
GF Food Banks	https://www.nationalceliac.org/the-gluten-free-food-bank
GIKids	https://www.gikids.org/content/3/en/celiac-disease
Gluten-Free Dietitian	https://www.glutenfreedietitian.com
Gluten Free Matzo	https://www.glutenfreematzo.com
Gluten in Medications	https://www.glutenfreedrugs.com
Gluten Intolerance Group	https://www.gluten.net
Low-gluten Altar Bread	https://www.altarbreadsbspa.com/altarbreads/low-gluten-breads
National Celiac Association	https://www.nationalceliac.org
National Institute of Diabetes and Digestive and Kidney Diseases	https://www.niddk.nih.gov
NIH	https://www.niddk.nih.gov/health-information/digestive-diseases/celiac-disease
National Library of Medicine	https://www.nlm.nih.gov/medlineplus/celiacdisease.html
North American Society For The Study of Celiac Disease	https://www.nasscd.org
Tricia Thompson, MS, RD Gluten Free Watchdog	https://www.glutenfreewatchdog.org
FDA	https://www.fda.gov/Food/Guidance Regulation/GuidanceDocumentsRegulatory Information/ucm059116.htm
USDA	https://www.nal.usda.gov/fnic/food-labeling

This list is not a comprehensive list and not a substitute for RDN consultation.

use and before eating. More research is needed on the gluten content of cosmetics, particularly of the lips (lipstick, lip balm) and hands (hand lotion), which are theoretically considered more suspect.[12] Over-the-counter and prescription medications and supplements may contain gluten as an excipient, filler, or capsule and, therefore need to be verified GF. Medications can be checked through reputable online sources (see **Table 2**) or a knowledgeable pharmacist. Nutritional supplements are regulated by the FDA, under FALCPA, and can be labeled GF.

CROSS-CONTACT

Cross-contact occurs when a GF food is exposed to a gluten-containing food, thus making it unsafe for a person with CD. Cross-contact can occur during growing, transportation, manufacturing, and food preparation in a restaurant, workplace, or in the home.

OATS

Although oats offer a great potential to increase the nutrient profile of the diet, the role of oats in a GFD has been controversial. Oats contain avenin, a protein that is similar to gluten. Oat sensitivity can present as an immune reaction to avenin, similar to gluten,[13] or as an intestinal reaction to the increased fiber content of the oats; this latter phenomenon can be found not just in CD but also in the general population.[14] Pure oats are naturally GF, but most are grown in or near barley, rye, and wheat. Oats can also be processed using the same equipment, which results in significant cross-contact, rendering them not suitable for individuals with CD.

In 2006, a growing and manufacturing process for GF oats was developed that is referred to as the purity protocol. The steps in the process include several precautions to avoid cross-contact, including dedicated equipment and facilities that do not share or process gluten-containing grains.[15]

For oats that have not been grown according to a purity protocol, companies have started using mechanical and optical sorting methods to "clean" oats. Special equipment is used to sort the oats from gluten-containing grains based on the differences in size, shape, density, texture, and color.[16] The need for proper, rigorous, stringent testing regardless of the type of oat is of utmost importance.[17] All oats consumed by patients with CD, at the very least, must be labeled GF.

Patients should discuss with their gastroenterologists and RDNs whether and when to include GF oats.[17] GF oat consumption should be limited to 50 to 60 g/d.[18] When GF oats are introduced into the diet, patients should be monitored closely for clinical or serologic evidence of adverse reactions.[18] Patients with severe disease should avoid oats altogether.[19]

ARSENIC AND THE GLUTEN-FREE DIET

Concern exists about the potential for increased arsenic and other heavy metal exposure[20] in both adult and pediatric populations caused by the high intake of rice-based products on the GFD.[20–22]

One study found higher levels of arsenic, mercury, and lead and lower levels of selenium, iron, copper, and zinc in rice and rice products versus wheat or nonrice GF grains.[23]

More research is needed to determine to what extent this exposure may present a long-term health risk to this population.[20,21] Clinicians should encourage consumption of a wide variety of whole GF grains[23] to minimize arsenic exposure and maximize micronutrient content.

WEIGHT CONCERNS OF THE GLUTEN-FREE DIET

Rates of overweight, obesity, and metabolic syndrome in CD[24,25] are expected to follow the worldwide upward trend in the general population.[26,27] Therefore, the GFD should be personalized to each patient addressing specific health issues. Although some health concerns exist about plant-based diets (bioavailability of nutrients, adequate vitamins and minerals, fatty acids), including vegan, vegetarian, and the Mediterranean diets, benefits include lower body weight, decreased risk of cancer, and a lower risk for ischemic heart disease.[28]

ALTERED WEIGHT IN CELIAC DISEASE

Overweight and obesity are increasingly common in the initial presentation of CD in adults[29–31] and have been documented in children.[32] A recent review study reported a 9% to 21% prevalence of overweight and a 0% to 6% prevalence of obesity in pediatric patients at diagnosis.[32]

Although the effect of the GFD on body mass index (BMI) of patients with newly diagnosed CD varies across studies,[26,33,34] overall patients tend to gain weight on a GFD.[6,25,35] Tortora and colleagues[25] reported an increased risk of metabolic syndrome 1 year after starting a GFD and a 4-fold increase in the risk for systemic hypertension in patients with CD. Although multiple factors influence BMI, weight gain in treated CD is likely caused by the increased nutrient absorption[25] coupled with the reliance on GF products. GF products frequently use refined flours and starches[36] and contain increased amounts of fat, sugar,[37] and salt compared with wheat-based products.[38]

Alternatively, continued weight loss on a GFD may be caused by nonadherence, refractory CD (RCD), inadequate caloric intake, or a healthier diet overall.[7] High-nutrition-risk patients may benefit from a GF enteral or oral feeding to provide adequate nutrition at diagnosis.[39] Celiac crisis, a life-threatening condition characterized by severe metabolic disturbances, malnutrition, and profuse diarrhea ,which often requires hospitalization and/or nutrition support, is not commonly seen in children or adults.[27,40,41] RDNs plays a key role in monitoring weight and modifying nutritional guidance accordingly.[29–31,33]

NUTRITIONAL DEFICIENCIES OF THE GLUTEN-FREE DIET

Compounding the risk of nutrient deficiency at diagnosis is the nutritional inadequacy of the traditional GFD.[30,36,37] In a study by Hallert and colleagues,[37] 37% of the participants showed signs of malnutrition with increased homocysteine levels despite endoscopic results indicating a healed small intestine. A subsequent study[30] revisited the nutritional deficiencies of long-term GFD-adherent participants with CD and found similar results.[37] In comparing the intake of the participants on a GFD with the general population controls, Hallert and colleagues[37] found that the number of bread servings was the same in both groups. However, the nutritional content of the GF bread was inferior to that of its wheat-based counterpart. In a 2005 study of standard GFD intake patterns, food records revealed deficiencies in B vitamins, fiber, calcium, and iron.[36] Women did not meet any of the recommended dietary standards and men only met the recommendation for iron. In an Italian study,[42] the overall caloric intake of participants with CD on a GFD was similar to that of the general population. However, when nutrient contents of the two diets were compared, the GFD was higher in fat, sugar, sweetened fruit juices, and simple carbohydrates.[42]

In a recent study of grain consumption patterns of individuals with CD on a GFD, 88% of adults and 83% of adolescents consumed ultraprocessed grains. Most grains consumed were brown rice and GF oats. Both adults and adolescents infrequently consumed alternative grains (quinoa, millet, buckwheat) and rarely as a whole grain.[43]

In a study by Lee and colleagues,[44] inclusion of alternative GF grains may be the solution to the nutritional deficit of the GFD. Similar to other studies, the typical intake of participants with CD relied heavily on prepared foods, processed quick and convenience products, and predominately white rice. In substituting only the grain portion of the diet with whole-grain brown rice, quinoa, and GF oats, the nutrient analysis was significantly improved ($P = .002$), with increases in key nutrients (fiber, folate, iron, and riboflavin) (**Fig. 1**).

DUAL DIAGNOSIS

Between 0.6% and 16% of patients with type 1 diabetes mellitus (T1DM) are affected by celiac disease at some point over their lifetimes.[45,46] The dietary management of CD and T1DM may add additional restrictions/limitations for patients. Most patients with T1DM present without gastrointestinal (GI) symptoms before a CD diagnosis, placing them at greater risk for noncompliance.[47]

Many manufactured GF products contain more refined carbohydrate, sugar, and fat, and less fiber per portion. Balancing healthy food choices, strict GFD, and diabetes may be difficult and affect compliance; these patients often require additional education and dietary surveillance.[46]

NUTRIENT DEFICIENCIES IN UNTREATED AND NEWLY DIAGNOSED CELIAC DISEASE

Nutritional deficiencies of macronutrients and micronutrients are frequently found in untreated or newly diagnosed CD (**Table 3**). The degree of malabsorption depends on the length of time before the celiac diagnosis and the degree of intestinal mucosal injury.[38] Anemia is common at diagnosis, caused by malabsorption of micronutrients, including iron, folic acid, and vitamin B_{12}, although not the only reason.[48,49]

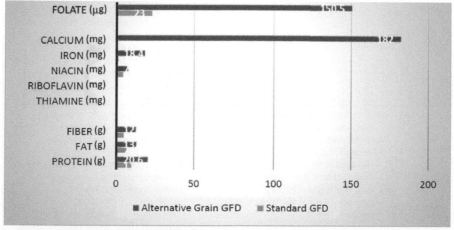

Fig. 1. Nutrient comparison of standard versus alternative grain GFD. (*From* Lee AR, Ng DL, Dave E, et al. The effect of substituting alternative grains in the diet on the nutritional profile of the gluten-free diet. J Hum Nutr Diet 2009;22(4):359–63; with permission.)

Table 3
Nutritional status, testing, and treatment of patients with celiac disease

Nutrient	Epidemiology and Nutritional Status at Diagnosis	Comments on Nutritional Testing and Treatment
Iron	28%–50% of patients are deficient at diagnosis[27,58] Common extraintestinal manifestation of CD[27]	Replete iron based on initial ferritin level[27] IV iron for severe symptomatic iron deficiency or oral intolerance[27,51] Iron deficiency anemia: • Daily MVM with iron or therapeutic iron dosing[8] Iron-rich foods: lean meats, seafood, nuts, beans, seeds, fortified GF cereals, leafy vegetables, dried fruit
Vitamin D	Vitamin D deficiency is common in CD[19] Much of the bone loss in CD is related to secondary hyperparathyroidism, which is probably caused by vitamin D deficiency and can only be partially reversed with a GFD[19] Deficiency caused by: • Villus atrophy and fat malabsorption[51] • Reduced intake of dairy caused by lactose intolerance[51,52] Deficiency partly responsible for low bone mineral density in untreated CD[6]; magnesium's role is also suggested[59]	No consensus about the optimal timing for DXA in CD, whether at diagnosis or during the follow-up[60] Meet vitamin D needs through foods enriched with vitamin D, as well as supplements, as needed[61] for adults with reduced bone density or reduced serum levels of 25-OHD[8] Vitamin D–rich foods: vitamin D–fortified cow's milk and milk substitutes, fatty fish (salmon, tuna, and mackerel)
Calcium	High rate of lactose intolerance in CD is a risk factor for increased risk of bone loss[60] See text for vitamin D epidemiology	RDN assesses intake[8] because serum calcium is not a good marker for calcium status[51] Calcium requirements vary by age[51] Recommend calcium supplementation if dietary calcium is inadequate,[52,62] suspected malabsorption, or low calcium serum levels[52] Advise adequate intake through food or supplement for adults with reduced bone density or reduced 25-OHD[8] See vitamin D re: DXA Calcium-rich foods: dairy (milk, yogurt, and cheese), fortified milk substitutes (soy, nut, pea), kale, broccoli
Vitamin B_{12}	8%–41% deficiency in newly diagnosed CD[27] Absorbed primarily in the ileum Reasons for B_{12} deficiency (although not well established) include: • Terminal ileal involvement likely[63] • Pancreatic insufficiency[64] • Competition for B_{12} by undesirable bacteria in SIBO[65]	Because of neurologic issues from untreated B_{12} deficiency check MMA in patients with low normal serum B_{12}[66] Consider parenteral vitamin B_{12} for severe deficiency, neurologic features, or ongoing malabsorption[66] Vitamin B_{12}–rich foods: animal products (fish, meat, poultry, dairy, and eggs), fortified GF cereals

(continued on next page)

Table 3 (*continued*)		
Nutrient	**Epidemiology and Nutritional Status at Diagnosis**	**Comments on Nutritional Testing and Treatment**
Folate	35%–49% of patients with CD may have low folate levels[66] Patients with CD with SIBO may have normal to increased serum folate levels[66]	RDN assesses intake and serum folate and makes dietary or supplementation recommendations[8] Check serum folate and recommend folate supplementation in women of childbearing age[66] Resolve B_{12} deficiency before folate supplementation is given[51,63] Folate-rich foods: liver, legumes, fortified GF cereals, peanuts, spinach, asparagus, broccoli, peas
Zinc	54%–67% deficiency in newly diagnosed CD[67] Most common deficiency of the trace elements[27]	No consensus on supplementation: • Supplement with zinc until serum level is normal[27] • Zinc levels can improve on the GFD with or without supplemental zinc[53] • After 1 year on a strict GFD, zinc deficiency resolves; long-term supplementation is typically not needed[51] Zinc-rich foods: oysters, red meat, poultry, beans, nuts, GF fortified cereals and dairy products
Vitamin B_6	14.5% deficiency in newly diagnosed CD[67] B_6 deficiency noted in 2 earlier pediatric celiac studies showing decreased pyridoxal phosphate in serum samples and duodenal mucosa[68,69]	Screen initially and monitor for symptoms or in the case of other B vitamin deficiencies[51] Caution MVM supplements may contain high levels of B_6 B_6-rich foods: chickpeas, liver, tuna, salmon, chicken, GF fortified cereals

Abbreviations: DXA, dual-energy X-ray absorptiometry; IV, intravenous; MMA, methylmalonic acid; MVM, multivitamin and mineral; 25-OHD, 25-hydroxyvitamin D; SIBO, small intestinal bacterial overgrowth.

Macrocytic anemia from folate or vitamin B_{12} deficiency can be difficult to uncover in patients with comorbid iron deficiency.[50]

Impaired intestinal mucosa can be associated with malabsorption of both macronutrients and micronutrients, including protein, calories, fat,[7] vitamin D,[51] calcium,[52] zinc,[53] copper,[27,54,55] carnitine,[56] and selenium.[49,57] At diagnosis, some patients benefit from a high-calorie, high-protein GFD.

NUTRITIONAL THERAPY AND NUTRIENT TESTING

At present the only treatment of CD is strict, lifelong adherence to the GFD. Individualized testing for newly diagnosed patients may include complete blood count,[41,66] iron status,[41,50] ferritin,[66] vitamin B_{12},[47] folate,[50,66] thyroid studies,[41] liver enzymes,[41] 25-hydroxyvitamin D,[41,50,66] calcium,[66] zinc,[41,50,66] copper,[66] magnesium,[19] carotene,[19] prothrombin time,[19] vitamin A,[19] vitamin E,[19] selenium,[19] B_6,[51]

B_1,[19] or other B vitamins.[51] No universal testing guidelines are in place for nutritional deficiencies in newly diagnosed CD.[7] Some investigators suggest that routine checking of fat-soluble vitamin levels may not be needed in children with CD[70]; others suggest checking vitamin D and vitamin A[71] (see **Table 3**).

There are no universal guidelines for supplementation.[7] Some individuals may require specific nutrient therapy until mucosal healing is complete.[27,38] Kelly and colleagues[50] suggest nutritional status should be monitored at the start of treatment with a GFD, every 3 to 6 months until normal, and then every 1 to 2 years. García-Manzanares and Lucendo[39] suggest following the World Health Organization's guidelines for the general population for daily intake of vitamins, minerals, water, and fiber. Wierdsma and colleagues[67] suggest a standard complete multivitamin supplement (100%–300% of recommended daily allowance) for newly diagnosed-patients. Some deficiencies continue years after initiation of the GFD.[37,72] Instead of long-term vitamin and mineral supplementation, Shepherd and Gibson[73] emphasize achieving nutritional adequacy from diet alone. The Academy of Nutrition and Dietetics recommends a GF age-specific and sex-specific multivitamin/mineral supplement only if the patient is unable to meet nutritional needs through diet.[8]

Oversupplementation of vitamins and minerals should be avoided.[74] RDNs should monitor intake, supplement use, and serologies and provide appropriate guidance. Nutritional supplements are regulated by the FDA and under FALCPA. Patients should only purchase multivitamins and other supplements that are labeled GF.

NUTRITION IN NONRESPONSIVE CELIAC DISEASE

Nonresponsive celiac disease (NRCD) affects ∼7%–30% of patients[6] with persistent symptoms and is a key reason for long-term follow-up.[75] After physician confirmation of CD,[6] an RDN assesses the intake for risk of chance gluten exposure and monitors the patient's celiac antibody levels because gluten is the most common culprit for continued symptoms.[76]

Additional causes of NRCD include, but are not limited to, small intestinal bacterial overgrowth (SIBO),[76,77] irritable bowel syndrome,[76,77] secondary lactose intolerance,[76,77] microscopic colitis,[50,76] disaccharide deficiency,[78] and, to a lesser extent, eating disorders, peptic ulcer disease, gastroparesis, Crohn disease, food allergies, common variable immune deficiency, duodenal adenocarcinoma,[76] pancreatic exocrine dysfunction,[46] cow's milk protein sensitivity,[77] and refractory CD (a rare, serious cause of NRCD).[76,79] The RDN has an integral role in the assessment and management of patients with all causes of NRCD to determine appropriate dietary interventions (**Table 4**).

GLUTEN CONTAMINATION ELIMINATION DIET

The gluten contamination elimination diet (GCED), is a temporary, strict, unprocessed foods diet protocol that can be used to differentiate between NRCD and RCD type 1 (see **Table 4**). The GCED can identify those patients who may be exposed to, and sensitive to, less gluten than is typically tolerated by most patients with CD.[96,97] Close monitoring by an RDN during the exclusion and carefully staged reintroduction phases is required.[96,97] In a trial of subjects who met criteria for RCD type 1, Hollon and colleagues[96] found the diagnosis was reversed in 83% of the subjects.

Table 4 Causes of nonresponsive celiac disease and dietary interventions	
Concerns	Nutrition Interventions
Secondary lactose intolerance	Presents in varying degrees with symptoms that mimic gluten exposure Some patients benefit initially from removal or reduction of lactose if symptoms are worsened by dairy[61] Calcium needs met through lactose-free or lactose-reduced products, and calcium-rich foods[8,36,80,81] and GF calcium supplements, when needed[8] Encourage vitamin D intake from dietary sources and supplementation, as needed[8,81]
IBS	~38% of patients with CD have IBS compared with 15%–20% in the general population[82] The low FODMAP diet, which temporarily reduces and rechallenges fermentable carbohydrates and sugar alcohol intake, is the accepted, evidence-based therapy for IBS[83] with varying success rates The temporary elimination/controlled reintroduction phases are carefully monitored by a skilled GI RDN to ensure patients meet nutritional needs and to provide a liberal, individualized, healthy diet for long-term symptom control[84] The low FODMAP diet has been found to be effective in controlling GI symptoms in CD[85]
SIBO	A common cause of persistent symptoms and can mimic gluten exposure[86] Weight loss, steatorrhea, malnutrition (eg, anemia), and other signs of malabsorption seen in more severe cases[87] Can result in normal to increased serum folate levels[66] Individualized dietary therapy: exclude lactose as needed[87]; reduce simple sugars[87,88]; increase fat for energy needs, as needed, using MCTs[87]; emphasize readily absorbed nutrients[88] Monitor weight and vitamin and mineral levels, particularly B_{12}, fat-soluble vitamins, calcium, and magnesium[65] The low FODMAP diet,[89] elemental diet,[89] and multifaceted integrative approaches, including herbal medications[89,90] as well as probiotics,[65,87,89,91] have been used to treat SIBO; more research is needed
MC	CD is found in 2%–20% of patients with MC[92] MC found in 4.3% of celiac cohort, a 70% increased risk compared with the general population[93] Dietary goal: improve patient's QOL and address symptoms; drug use, excess use of caffeine, alcohol, and dairy products may exacerbate MC[92]
Food allergy	Requires specific allergy testing followed by removal of the allergen and, when appropriate, a supervised oral challenge
RCD	Monitor to exclude possible gluten contamination[6] Focus on nutritional assessment and support as the initial therapy in RCD[94] Fluid, electrolytes, and acid-base balance should be assessed and managed as a priority, especially in the presence of severe malabsorption, weight loss, muscle wasting, and edema Complete blood count, vitamin B_{12}, folate, albumin, calcium, and vitamin D levels should also be measured and corrected Oral supplements should be encouraged and MCTs can be used to boost calorie intake In the presence of severe malnutrition, total parenteral nutrition should be initiated and a more thorough search made for fat-soluble vitamin, mineral, and trace element deficiencies[94] The elemental diet may be considered as a therapeutic option in type 1 RCD[95]

Abbreviations: FODMAP, fermentable oligosaccharides, disaccharides, monosaccharides and polyols; IBS, irritable bowel syndrome; MC, microscopic colitis; MCTs, medium-chain triglycerides.

IMPACT ON QUALITY OF LIFE

Many domains of an individual's QOL are affected by their physical health, presence of symptoms, treatment burden, prognosis, and perception of their own health. It must be recognized that the GFD affects all aspects of life, including culture, social, and emotional needs, and that eating encompasses more than just meeting the physiologic need for nutrients. Studies have reported poor QOL scores for individuals with CD, caused by a statistically significant burden of the disease from multiple factors, including cost, restrictive nature of the diet, and emotional loss. The RDN assesses the psychological impact of the diet and disease and develops strategies with the patient to navigate successfully.

The cost of the GFD negatively affects the QOL of individuals with CD. In a study by Lee and colleagues,[98] the cost of GF foods was 240% more than their wheat-based counterparts (**Fig. 2**).

Several studies have described the interrelationship between the rigid nature of the GFD, dietary compliance, and QOL scores.[99–102] Several studies describe increased anxiety associated with social occasions.[101–103] Seventy-four percent of participants (n = 788) reported anxiety and depression compared with only 50% before diagnosis.[103] Fear and anxiety are often associated with socializing with friends, being different, and fear of contamination of food.[99–101] The GFD has been reported to negatively affect the social domain of QOL. According to the study by Cranney and collegues,[100] 81% of respondents avoid restaurants, 38% avoid travel, and 91% bring their own GF food when traveling.

In the study by Lee and colleagues,[102] 45% of participants reported that their physical health affected interactions with family, friends, or social groups versus 21% of controls. Individuals with CD are significantly negatively affected (P<.0001) in the areas of social activities with family, friends, or groups (**Fig. 3**).[102]

In a recent QOL study, not only was the overall QOL score higher than in previous studies but subjects with social support had the highest QOL scores. Of the 42% reporting use of social support networks (online 17.9%, face to face 10.8%, or both 12.8%), QOL scores were higher for those individuals who used only face-to-face social support versus only online support (72.6 vs 66.7; P<.0001). A longer duration of face-to-face social support use was associated with higher QOL scores (P<.0005).

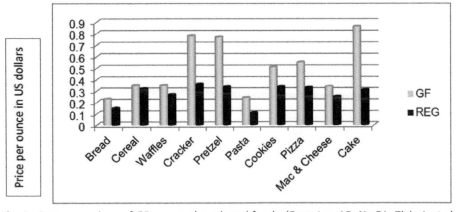

Fig. 2. Cost comparison of GF versus wheat-based foods. (*From* Lee AR, Ng DL, Zivin J, et al. Economic burden of a gluten-free diet. J Hum Nutr Diet 2007;20(5):423–30; with permission.)

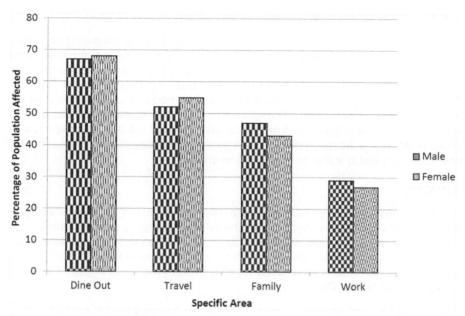

Fig. 3. Negative impact of GFD on QOL by specific area and gender. (*From* Lee AR, Ng DL, Diamond B, et al. Living with coeliac disease: survey results from the U.S.A. J Hum Nutr Diet 2012;25(3):233–8; with permission.)

By contrast, a longer duration and increased frequency of online social support use was associated with lower QOL scores ($P<.03$).[104]

PSYCHOLOGICAL ASPECTS OF RESTRICTIVE DIETS

Researchers are now investigating whether diminished QOL in CD has farther reaching impacts, including psychological aspects, eating disorders, and association with depression.[105,106] In a multicenter study,[106] female adolescents with CD and a comorbid eating disorder had higher rates of depression and dietary noncompliance. There were no differences found in coping mechanisms between the groups with and without eating disorder in addition to their CD. A study evaluating the association between CD and presence of other psychological disorders[105] found a higher rate of major depressive disorder in individuals with CD compared with controls (30.0% vs 8.3%, $P<.0001$). Similar results were found when panic disorder and bipolar disorder were investigated (18.3% vs 5.4%, $P<.001$; and 4.3% vs 0.4%, $P<.005$) respectively. The investigators strongly suggest screening for CD in individuals with affective disorders as well as screening for these disorders in the celiac population.[105]

An increased frequency of altered eating habits was found in a study of patients with untreated CD compared with healthy controls.[107,108] The investigators concluded the increased frequency of disordered eating was multifactorial, a potential result of altered psychological status associated with CD, presence of GI symptoms, and the focus on high-carbohydrate food intake before diagnosis.[108] Assessment of the effect of a restrictive diet such as insulin-dependent diabetes and/or GFD shows that these individuals show a variety of cognitive, emotional, and behavioral changes.[107] In several of these patient groups, individuals on a restrictive diet were more likely to experience episodes of overeating and binge eating. Thus, the psychological burden of a restrictive diet further affects individuals' QOL.

SCHOOL ACCOMMODATION

Of special concern to parents of school-aged children with CD is navigating the school cafeteria, trips, and classroom events. Although many schools have responded to the increased requests for safe spaces from parents of children with nut allergies, the same has not been the case with regard to the GFD. The Americans with Disability Act allows parents to request an individual 504 accommodation plan for their children, a legally binding document providing full participation in all of the school's academic, social, and physical activities and programs safely without risk of gluten exposure or social isolation. It is the responsibility of the parents to collaborate with their school to develop a plan that is suited to the individual child.[109]

SUMMARY

Nutrition counseling with an RDN is vital for the assessment of the patient's acceptance of the diagnosis and adoption of the GFD. Together, a comprehensive plan will be developed to guide the patient with appropriate nutrition recommendations, resources, and support (see **Table 2**). The study by Lee and colleagues[104] confirms the original NIH guidance of comprehensive nutrition counseling by an expert RDN as the key to the treatment of CD.

DISCLOSURE

M. Dennis has published 1 book and several peer-reviewed journal articles related to CD and founded and owns a nutritional consulting business, Delete the Wheat. She is Senior Nutrition Consultant for the National Celiac Association, Low FODMAP diet advisory board for University of Monash Australia. A.R. Lee has published several peer-reviewed journal articles related to CD, the GFD, and QOL. She is on the medical advisory board for Schar, a GF food company, and editor for UpToDate's section on pediatric CD. T. McCarthy founded and owns a nutritional consulting business, Tara McCarthy RD. She is currently working as a consultant in a study with a company called the Gluten Detective.

REFERENCES

1. Rubio-Tapia A, Ludvigsson JF, Brantner TL, et al. The prevalence of celiac disease in the United States. Am J Gastroenterol 2012;107(10):1538–44 [quiz: 1537, 1545].
2. Fasano A, Berti I, Gerarduzzi T, et al. Prevalence of celiac disease in at-risk and not-at-risk groups in the United States: a large multicenter study. Arch Intern Med 2003;163(3):286–92.
3. Reilly NR. The gluten-free diet: recognizing fact, fiction, and fad. J Pediatr 2016; 175:206–10.
4. Tanpowpong P, Broder-Fingert S, Katz AJ, et al. Predictors of gluten avoidance and implementation of a gluten-free diet in children and adolescents without confirmed celiac disease. J Pediatr 2012;161(3):471–5.
5. National Institutes of Health Consensus Development Conference Statement. 2004. Available at: https://consensus.nih.gov/2004/2004CeliacDisease118html. htm. Accessed April 25, 2018.
6. Rubio-Tapia A, Hill ID, Kelly CP, et al. ACG clinical guidelines: diagnosis and management of celiac disease. Am J Gastroenterol 2013;108(5):656–76 [quiz: 677].

7. See J, Murray JA. Gluten-free diet: the medical and nutrition management of celiac disease. Nutr Clin Pract 2006;21(1):1–15.
8. Dennis M, Kupper C, Lee AR, et al. Celiac disease toolkit. American Dietetic Association; 2011. Available at: https://www.eatrightpro.org/research.
9. Questions and answers: gluten-free food labeling final rule. 2017. Available at: https://www.fda.gov/Food/GuidanceRegulation/GuidanceDocumentsRegulatory Information/Allergens/ucm362880.htm. Accessed May 10, 2018.
10. Gluten and food labeling. 2018. Available at: https://www.fda.gov/Food/ GuidanceRegulation/GuidanceDocumentsRegulatoryInformation/Allergens/ ucm367654.htm. Accessed June 1, 2018.
11. Food labeling fact sheets. Available at: https://www.fsis.usda.gov/wps/portal/ fsis/topics/food-safety-education/get-answers/food-safety-fact-sheets/food-labeling. Accessed May 30, 2018.
12. Thompson T, Grace T. Gluten in cosmetics: is there a reason for concern? J Acad Nutr Diet 2012;112(9):1316–23.
13. Arentz-Hansen H, Fleckenstein B, Molberg Ø, et al. The molecular basis for oat intolerance in patients with celiac disease. PLoS Med 2004;1(1):e1.
14. Gilissen LJWJ, van der Meer IM, Smulders MJM. Why oats are safe and healthy for celiac disease patients. Med Sci (Basel) 2016;4(4). https://doi.org/10.3390/ medsci4040021.
15. Allred L, Kupper C, Iverson G, et al. Definition of the "purity protocol" for producing gluten-free oats. Cereal Chem 94(3). Available at: https://doi.org/10.1094/ CCHEM-01-17-0017-VO. Accessed May 31, 2018.
16. Harmond J, Brandenburg N, Klein L. Mechanical seed cleaning and handling. 1968. Available at: https://naldc.nal.usda.gov/download/CAT87208718/PDF. Accessed May 30, 2018.
17. NASSCD releases summary statement on oats. 2016. Available at: https://celiac. org/blog/2016/04/nasscd-releases-summary-statement-on-oats. Accessed May 30, 2018.
18. Aaltonen K, Laurikka P, Huhtala H, et al. The long-term consumption of oats in celiac disease patients is safe: a large cross-sectional study. Nutrients 2017; 9(6). https://doi.org/10.3390/nu9060611.
19. Ciclitira PJ. Management of celiac disease in adults. 2017. Available at: https:// www.uptodate.com/contents/management-of-celiac-disease-in-adults?topicRef= 1999&source=see_link. Accessed May 19, 2018.
20. Raehsler SL, Choung RS, Marietta EV, et al. Accumulation of heavy metals in people on a gluten-free diet. Clin Gastroenterol Hepatol 2018;16(2):244–51.
21. Munera-Picazo S, Ramírez-Gandolfo A, Burló F, et al. Inorganic and total arsenic contents in rice-based foods for children with celiac disease. J Food Sci 2014; 79(1):T122–8.
22. Munera-Picazo S, Burló F, Carbonell-Barrachina ÁA. Arsenic speciation in rice-based food for adults with celiac disease. Food Addit Contam Part A Chem Anal Control Expo Risk Assess 2014;31(8):1358–66.
23. Punshon T, Jackson BP. Essential micronutrient and toxic trace element concentrations in gluten containing and gluten-free foods. Food Chem 2018;252: 258–64.
24. Ogden CL, Carroll MD, Fryar CD, et al. Prevalence of obesity among adults and youth: United States, 2011-2014. NCHS Data Brief 2015;(219):1–8.
25. Tortora R, Capone P, De Stefano G, et al. Metabolic syndrome in patients with coeliac disease on a gluten-free diet. Aliment Pharmacol Ther 2015;41(4): 352–9.

26. Ukkola A, Mäki M, Kurppa K, et al. Changes in body mass index on a gluten-free diet in coeliac disease: a nationwide study. Eur J Intern Med 2012;23(4):384–8.
27. Theethira TG, Dennis M, Leffler DA. Nutritional consequences of celiac disease and the gluten-free diet. Expert Rev Gastroenterol Hepatol 2014;8(2):123–9.
28. Tuso PJ, Ismail MH, Ha BP, et al. Nutritional update for physicians: plant-based diets. Perm J 2013;17(2):61–6.
29. Tucker E, Rostami K, Prabhakaran S, et al. Patients with coeliac disease are increasingly overweight or obese on presentation. J Gastrointestin Liver Dis 2012;21(1):11–5.
30. Dickey W, Kearney N. Overweight in celiac disease: prevalence, clinical characteristics, and effect of a gluten-free diet. Am J Gastroenterol 2006;101(10): 2356–9.
31. Sonti R, Green PHR. Celiac disease: obesity in celiac disease. Nat Rev Gastroenterol Hepatol 2012;9(5):247–8.
32. Diamanti A, Capriati T, Basso MS, et al. Celiac disease and overweight in children: an update. Nutrients 2014;6(1):207–20.
33. Kabbani TA, Goldberg A, Kelly CP, et al. Body mass index and the risk of obesity in coeliac disease treated with the gluten-free diet. Aliment Pharmacol Ther 2012;35(6):723–9.
34. Cheng J, Brar PS, Lee AR, et al. Body mass index in celiac disease: beneficial effect of a gluten-free diet. J Clin Gastroenterol 2010;44(4):267–71.
35. Mohsen Dehghani S, Ostovar S, Ataollahi M, et al. The effect of gluten-free diet among celiac patients aged 3-12 years old on BMI during 2006 to 2014 at Nemazee Teaching hospital. Rev Gastroenterol Peru 2017;37(4):323–8.
36. Thompson T, Dennis M, Higgins LA, et al. Gluten-free diet survey: are Americans with coeliac disease consuming recommended amounts of fibre, iron, calcium and grain foods? J Hum Nutr Diet 2005;18(3):163–9.
37. Hallert C, Grant C, Grehn S, et al. Evidence of poor vitamin status in coeliac patients on a gluten-free diet for 10 years. Aliment Pharmacol Ther 2002;16(7): 1333–9.
38. Saturni L, Ferretti G, Bacchetti T. The gluten-free diet: safety and nutritional quality. Nutrients 2010;2(1):16–34.
39. García-Manzanares A, Lucendo AJ. Nutritional and dietary aspects of celiac disease. Nutr Clin Pract 2011;26(2):163–73.
40. Jamma S, Rubio-Tapia A, Kelly CP, et al. Celiac crisis is a rare but serious complication of celiac disease in adults. Clin Gastroenterol Hepatol 2010;8(7): 587–90.
41. Leffler DA, Dennis M, Kelly CP. Celiac disease. In: Podolsky DK, Camilleri M, Fitz JG, Kalloo AN, Shanahan F, Wang TC, editors. Yamada textbook of gastroenterology. CHAPTER 64, Celiac Disease. Rochester (United Kingdom): PM Book Publishing; 2015. p. 1264–75.
42. Zuccotti G, Fabiano V, Dilillo D, et al. Intakes of nutrients in Italian children with celiac disease and the role of commercially available gluten-free products. J Hum Nutr Diet 2013;26(5):436–44.
43. Lee AR, Wolf R, Lebwohl B, et al. Alternative grain intake among adults with celiac disease: a prospective study. Gastroenterology 154(6):S-493–4.
44. Lee AR, Ng DL, Dave E, et al. The effect of substituting alternative grains in the diet on the nutritional profile of the gluten-free diet. J Hum Nutr Diet 2009;22(4): 359–63.
45. Rewers M, Liu E, Simmons J, et al. Celiac disease associated with type 1 diabetes mellitus. Endocrinol Metab Clin North Am 2004;33(1):197–214, xi.

46. Scaramuzza AE, Mantegazza C, Bosetti A, et al. Type 1 diabetes and celiac disease: the effects of gluten free diet on metabolic control. World J Diabetes 2013; 4(4):130–4.
47. Mahmud FH, Murray JA, Kudva YC, et al. Celiac disease in type 1 diabetes mellitus in a North American community: prevalence, serologic screening, and clinical features. Mayo Clin Proc 2005;80(11):1429–34.
48. Harper JW, Holleran SF, Ramakrishnan R, et al. Anemia in celiac disease is multifactorial in etiology. Am J Hematol 2007;82(11):996–1000.
49. Halfdanarson TR, Litzow MR, Murray JA. Hematologic manifestations of celiac disease. Blood 2007;109(2):412–21.
50. Kelly CP, Bai JC, Liu E, et al. Advances in diagnosis and management of celiac disease. Gastroenterology 2015;148(6):1175–86.
51. Naik RD, Seidner DL, Adams DW. Nutritional consideration in celiac disease and nonceliac gluten sensitivity. Gastroenterol Clin North Am 2018;47(1):139–54.
52. Corazza GR, Di Stefano M, Mauriño E, et al. Bones in coeliac disease: diagnosis and treatment. Best Pract Res Clin Gastroenterol 2005;19(3):453–65.
53. Rawal P, Thapa BR, Prasad R, et al. Zinc supplementation to patients with celiac disease–is it required? J Trop Pediatr 2010;56(6):391–7.
54. Goodman BP, Mistry DH, Pasha SF, et al. Copper deficiency myeloneuropathy due to occult celiac disease. Neurologist 2009;15(6):355–6.
55. Botero-López JE, Araya M, Parada A, et al. Micronutrient deficiencies in patients with typical and atypical celiac disease. J Pediatr Gastroenterol Nutr 2011;53(3): 265–70.
56. Lerner A, Gruener N, Iancu TC. Serum carnitine concentrations in coeliac disease. Gut 1993;34(7):933–5.
57. Stazi AV, Trinti B. Selenium deficiency in celiac disease: risk of autoimmune thyroid diseases. Minerva Med 2008;99(6):643–53 [in Italian].
58. Grisolano SW, Oxentenko AS, Murray JA, et al. The usefulness of routine small bowel biopsies in evaluation of iron deficiency anemia. J Clin Gastroenterol 2004;38(9):756–60.
59. Rude RK, Olerich M. Magnesium deficiency: possible role in osteoporosis associated with gluten-sensitive enteropathy. Osteoporos Int 1996;6(6):453–61.
60. Bianchi M-L, Bardella MT. Bone in celiac disease. Osteoporos Int 2008;19(12): 1705–16.
61. Kelly CP, Dennis M. Patient education: celiac disease in adults (beyond the basics). 2015. Available at: https://www.uptodate.com/contents/celiac-disease-in-adults-beyond-the-basics?topicRef=15378&source=see_link. Accessed May 30, 2018
62. Zanchetta MB, Longobardi V, Bai JC. Bone and celiac disease. Curr Osteoporos Rep 2016;14(2):43–8.
63. Dahele A, Ghosh S. Vitamin B12 deficiency in untreated celiac disease. Am J Gastroenterol 2001;96(3):745–50.
64. Hjelt K. The role of the exocrine pancreas in early-onset vitamin B12 malabsorption in gluten-challenged celiac children. J Pediatr Gastroenterol Nutr 1991; 13(1):27–31.
65. Dukowicz AC, Lacy BE, Levine GM. Small intestinal bacterial overgrowth: a comprehensive review. Gastroenterol Hepatol (N Y) 2007;3(2):112–22.
66. Oxentenko AS, Murray JA. Celiac disease: ten things that every gastroenterologist should know. Clin Gastroenterol Hepatol 2015;13(8):1396–404 [quiz: e127–9].

67. Wierdsma NJ, van Bokhorst-de van der Schueren MAE, Berkenpas M, et al. Vitamin and mineral deficiencies are highly prevalent in newly diagnosed celiac disease patients. Nutrients 2013;5(10):3975–92.

68. Reinken L, Zieglauer H. Vitamin B-6 absorption in children with acute celiac disease and in control subjects. J Nutr 1978;108(10):1562–5.

69. Reinken L, Zieglauer H, Berger H. Vitamin B6 nutriture of children with acute celiac disease, celiac disease in remission, and of children with normal duodenal mucosa. Am J Clin Nutr 1976;29(7):750–3.

70. Imam MH, Ghazzawi Y, Murray JA, et al. Is it necessary to assess for fat-soluble vitamin deficiencies in pediatric patients with newly diagnosed celiac disease? J Pediatr Gastroenterol Nutr 2014;59(2):225–8.

71. Tokgöz Y, Terlemez S, Karul A. Fat soluble vitamin levels in children with newly diagnosed celiac disease, a case control study. BMC Pediatr 2018;18(1):130.

72. Hallert C, Svensson M, Tholstrup J, et al. Clinical trial: B vitamins improve health in patients with coeliac disease living on a gluten-free diet. Aliment Pharmacol Ther 2009;29(8):811–6.

73. Shepherd SJ, Gibson PR. Nutritional inadequacies of the gluten-free diet in both recently-diagnosed and long-term patients with coeliac disease. J Hum Nutr Diet 2013;26(4):349–58.

74. Reguła J, Smidowicz A. Share of dietary supplements in nutrition of coeliac disease patients. Acta Sci Pol Technol Aliment 2014;13(3):301–7.

75. Silvester JA, Graff LA, Rigaux L, et al. Symptoms of functional intestinal disorders are common in patients with celiac disease following transition to a gluten-free diet. Dig Dis Sci 2017;62(9):2449–54.

76. Leffler DA, Dennis M, Hyett B, et al. Etiologies and predictors of diagnosis in nonresponsive celiac disease. Clin Gastroenterol Hepatol 2007;5(4):445–50.

77. Ludvigsson JF, Bai JC, Biagi F, et al. Diagnosis and management of adult coeliac disease: guidelines from the British Society of Gastroenterology. Gut 2014;63(8):1210–28.

78. Fine K, Meyer R, Lee E. The prevalence and causes of chronic diarrhea in patients with celiac sprue treated with a gluten-free diet. Gastroenterology 1997; 112(6):1830–8.

79. Abdulkarim AS, Burgart LJ, See J, et al. Etiology of nonresponsive celiac disease: results of a systematic approach. Am J Gastroenterol 2002;97(8): 2016–21.

80. Schuppan D, Dennis MD, Kelly CP. Celiac disease: epidemiology, pathogenesis, diagnosis, and nutritional management. Nutr Clin Care 2005;8(2):54–69.

81. Theethira TG, Dennis M. Celiac disease and the gluten-free diet: consequences and recommendations for improvement. Dig Dis 2015;33(2):175–82.

82. Sainsbury A, Sanders DS, Ford AC. Prevalence of irritable bowel syndrome-type symptoms in patients with celiac disease: a meta-analysis. Clin Gastroenterol Hepatol 2013;11(4):359–65.e1.

83. Harvie RM, Chisholm AW, Bisanz JE, et al. Long-term irritable bowel syndrome symptom control with reintroduction of selected FODMAPs. World J Gastroenterol 2017;23(25):4632–43.

84. O'Keeffe M, Jansen C, Martin L, et al. Long-term impact of the low-FODMAP diet on gastrointestinal symptoms, dietary intake, patient acceptability, and healthcare utilization in irritable bowel syndrome. Neurogastroenterol Motil 2018; 30(1). https://doi.org/10.1111/nmo.13154.

85. Testa A, Imperatore N, Rispo A, et al. Beyond irritable bowel syndrome: the efficacy of the low Fodmap diet for improving symptoms in inflammatory bowel

diseases and celiac disease. Dig Dis 2018;1–10. https://doi.org/10.1159/000489487.

86. Tursi A, Brandimarte G, Giorgetti G. High prevalence of small intestinal bacterial overgrowth in celiac patients with persistence of gastrointestinal symptoms after gluten withdrawal. Am J Gastroenterol 2003;98(4):839–43.

87. Bures J, Cyrany J, Kohoutova D, et al. Small intestinal bacterial overgrowth syndrome. World J Gastroenterol 2010;16(24):2978–90.

88. Salem A, Roland B. Small intestinal bacterial overgrowth (SIBO). J Gastrointest Dig Syst 2014;4(5):1–6.

89. Rezaie A, Pimentel M, Rao SS. How to test and treat small intestinal bacterial overgrowth: an evidence-based approach. Curr Gastroenterol Rep 2016;18(2):8.

90. Kwiatkowski L, Rice E, Langland J. Integrative treatment of chronic abdominal bloating and pain associated with overgrowth of small intestinal bacteria: a case report. Altern Ther Health Med 2017;23(4):56–61.

91. Zhong C, Qu C, Wang B, et al. Probiotics for preventing and treating small intestinal bacterial overgrowth: a meta-analysis and systematic review of current evidence. J Clin Gastroenterol 2017;51(4):300–11.

92. Bohr J, Wickbom A, Hegedus A, et al. Diagnosis and management of microscopic colitis: current perspectives. Clin Exp Gastroenterol 2014;7:273–84.

93. Green PHR, Yang J, Cheng J, et al. An association between microscopic colitis and celiac disease. Clin Gastroenterol Hepatol 2009;7(11):1210–6.

94. Abdallah H, Leffler D, Dennis M, et al. Refractory celiac disease. Curr Gastroenterol Rep 2007;9(5):401–5.

95. Olaussen RW, Løvik A, Tollefsen S, et al. Effect of elemental diet on mucosal immunopathology and clinical symptoms in type 1 refractory celiac disease. Clin Gastroenterol Hepatol 2005;3(9):875–85.

96. Hollon JR, Cureton PA, Martin ML, et al. Trace gluten contamination may play a role in mucosal and clinical recovery in a subgroup of diet-adherent non-responsive celiac disease patients. BMC Gastroenterol 2013;13:40.

97. Leonard MM, Cureton P, Fasano A. Indications and use of the gluten contamination elimination diet for patients with non-responsive celiac disease. Nutrients 2017;9(10). https://doi.org/10.3390/nu9101129.

98. Lee AR, Ng DL, Zivin J, et al. Economic burden of a gluten-free diet. J Hum Nutr Diet 2007;20(5):423–30.

99. Ciacci C, Iavarone A, Siniscalchi M, et al. Psychological dimensions of celiac disease: toward an integrated approach. Dig Dis Sci 2002;47(9):2082–7.

100. Cranney A, Zarkadas M, Graham ID, et al. The Canadian Celiac Health Survey. Dig Dis Sci 2007;52(4):1087–95.

101. Johnston SD, Rodgers C, Watson RG. Quality of life in screen-detected and typical coeliac disease and the effect of excluding dietary gluten. Eur J Gastroenterol Hepatol 2004;16(12):1281–6.

102. Lee AR, Ng DL, Diamond B, et al. Living with coeliac disease: survey results from the U.S.A. J Hum Nutr Diet 2012;25(3):233–8.

103. Gray AM, Papanicolas IN. Impact of symptoms on quality of life before and after diagnosis of coeliac disease: results from a UK population survey. BMC Health Serv Res 2010;10:105.

104. Lee AR, Wolf R, Contento I, et al. Coeliac disease: the association between quality of life and social support network participation. J Hum Nutr Diet 2016;29(3):383–90.

105. Rocha S, Gandolfi L, Santos JE. The psychosocial impacts caused by diagnosis and treatment of coeliac disease. Rev Esc Enferm USP 2016;50(1):66–72.
106. Wagner G, Zeiler M, Berger G, et al. Eating disorders in adolescents with celiac disease: influence of personality characteristics and coping. Eur Eat Disord Rev 2015;23(5):361–70.
107. Polivy J. Psychological consequences of food restriction. J Am Diet Assoc 1996; 96(6):589–92 [quiz: 593–4].
108. Passananti V, Siniscalchi M, Zingone F, et al. Prevalence of eating disorders in adults with celiac disease. Gastroenterol Res Pract 2013;2013:491657.
109. Parent and educator resource guide to section 504 in public elementary and secondary schools. 2016. Available at: https://www2.ed.gov/about/offices/list/ocr/docs/504-resource-guide-201612.pdf. Accessed May 31, 2018.

Capsule Endoscopy and Enteroscopy in Celiac Disease

Suzanne K. Lewis, MD[a],*, Carol E. Semrad, MD[b]

KEYWORDS

- Celiac disease • Capsule endoscopy • VCE • Enteroscopy
- Device-assisted enteroscopy • Refractory celiac disease

KEY POINTS

- Capsule endoscopy is a well-tolerated, safe method to examine the small intestine, and is more sensitive than standard endoscopy to detect villus atrophy.
- Capsule endoscopy can assist in diagnosing Celiac disease for patients unable to have an endoscopy for duodenal biopsy and in cases of equivocal diagnosis.
- Capsule endoscopy and enteroscopy, in combination with radiographic enterography, are of proven benefit in the evaluation of complicated celiac disease especially refractory celiac disease type II.
- Limitations of video capsule endoscopy include the inability to obtain tissue diagnosis, subjective interpretation, possible capsule retention, and incomplete examinations.
- Computer-assisted programs to detect villus atrophy and capsule and enteroscopy design advances are in development.

INTRODUCTION

Video capsule endoscopy (VCE) is a minimally invasive examination that produces highly magnified views of the entire small bowel mucosa. It was introduced in 2001 and has revolutionized the diagnosis and management of small bowel diseases, including obscure gastrointestinal bleeding, small bowel Crohn's disease, other ulcerating diseases, polyposis syndromes, small bowel tumors, and complicated celiac disease.[1] The role of VCE in celiac disease is still evolving. The advantage over standard endoscopy is the highly magnified view of the mucosa for better detection of villus changes. There is also the ability to examine the entire small bowel mucosa that

Disclosure: No disclosures.
[a] Division of Digestive Diseases, Celiac Disease Center at Columbia University, Columbia University, 180 Fort Washington Avenue, New York, NY 10032, USA; [b] The University of Chicago, 5841 South Maryland Avenue, MC 4080 S401, Chicago, IL 60637, USA
* Corresponding author.
E-mail address: skl3@cumc.columbia.edu

Gastroenterol Clin N Am 48 (2019) 73–84
https://doi.org/10.1016/j.gtc.2018.09.005

may be useful in cases of patchy villus atrophy. The main value is to detect complications in patients with celiac disease who have recurrent, persistent, or worrisome symptoms.

Duodenal biopsy is the gold standard for the diagnosis of celiac disease,[2] but it is not perfect. Villus atrophy can be patchy leading to false-negative results, or can be more distal than the duodenum and not reached by standard upper endoscopy, and therefore missed on biopsy.[3–6] Endoscopists may not obtain the recommended 4 to 6 biopsies during upper endoscopy, limiting diagnostic yield.[7] There is also variability in the interpretation of celiac histology such as in community hospitals or some commercial laboratories that may not consistently recognize the features of celiac disease.[8] Interpretation of the biopsies can also be affected by poor orientation. Endoscopy is invasive and may not be acceptable to patients owing to significant comorbidity or fear of the procedure. It involves anesthesia and days missed from school or work. In some cases, endoscopy with biopsies may be contraindicated owing to underlying medical conditions, such as significant cardiopulmonary disease and bleeding disorders.

The advantage of VCE is that it is minimally invasive, relatively safe,[9] and provides a high-resolution 8-fold magnification of the mucosa, similar to that of the dissection microscope.[10] In contrast with conventional endoscopy, the VCE examination is done without the use of air insufflation and the capsule is propelled distally by the normal peristalsis of the gastrointestinal tract. The capsule provides excellent visualization of the villus pattern (**Fig. 1**).

INDICATIONS FOR VIDEO CAPSULE ENDOSCOPY IN CELIAC DISEASE

There have been several guidelines proposed for the use of capsule endoscopy in celiac disease. An international consensus conference in 2005[11] advised that VCE can be considered in the evaluation of known or suspected celiac disease in certain circumstances, such as when a patient has positive serology and suspected celiac disease but is unable or unwilling to have a conventional endoscopy. It can be considered in cases of positive celiac serology (tissue transglutaminase or endomysial antibody (EMA)) and normal duodenal histology to examine more distal parts of the small bowel for villus atrophy. VCE is indicated in patients with celiac disease who develop warning signs such as anemia, weight loss, and gastrointestinal bleeding, and in those with

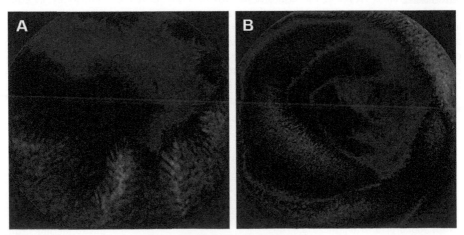

Fig. 1. (*A*) Normal villi example 1. (*B*) Normal villi example 2.

refractory celiac disease, especially type II, to evaluate for malignancy and other complications such as ulcerative jejunitis. In those with refractory celiac disease or suspected malignancy, VCE in combination with endoscopy, colonoscopy, and radiographic enterography followed by device-assisted enteroscopy may be required. The European Society of Gastrointestinal Endoscopy clinical guidelines, published in 2015,[12] concur with these recommendations. There is some disagreement as to the use of VCE for suspected celiac disease, particularly in the setting of a positive celiac disease serology and normal duodenal biopsy.[13]

Mucosal changes of celiac disease seen on upper endoscopy include scalloping of the mucosal folds, micronodularity, fissuring or mosaic pattern, and reduced duodenal folds,[14,15] changes readily identified on capsule endoscopy[16,17] (**Fig. 2**). VCE has excellent accuracy in identifying villus atrophy. Petroniene and colleagues[16] compared 10 patients with Marsh 3 histology with controls, and reported that VCE when compared with endoscopy was 100% specific, and tended toward a better sensitivity than endoscopy (70% vs 60%). There was a positive predictive value of 100% and a negative predictive value of 77%. Other studies have shown that VCE is more sensitive than optical endoscopy for detecting villus atrophy. In a study of 35 patients with villus atrophy, Murray and colleagues[3] found that VCE had a better

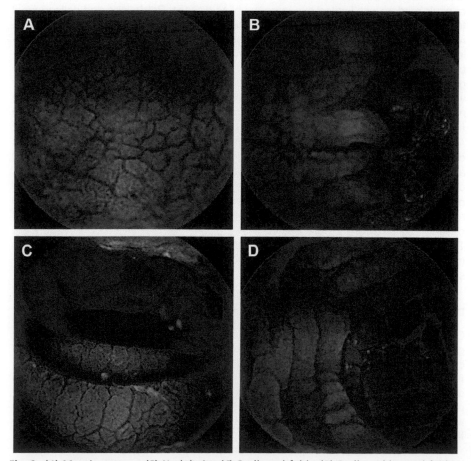

Fig. 2. (*A*) Mosaic pattern. (*B*) Nodularity. (*C*) Scalloped folds. (*D*) Scalloped layered folds.

sensitivity as compared with conventional endoscopy (92% vs 55%; $P = .0005$; specificity, 100%). In a study of 43 patients by Rondonotti and colleagues,[18] capsule endoscopy as compared with the gold standard of duodenal biopsy showed a sensitivity of 87.5%, specificity of 90.9%, positive predictive value of 96.5%, and negative predictive value of 71.4%. In a metaanalysis[19] of studies to determine the accuracy of VCE in celiac disease, a total of 166 patients from 6 studies were evaluated. The overall pooled VCE sensitivity was 89% (95% confidence interval, 82%–94%), and specificity 95% (95% confidence interval, 89%–98%).

When signs of villus atrophy are seen on VCE, there is a high probability that the patient has celiac disease; however, a normal capsule study does not exclude celiac disease. Biagi and colleagues[20] studied 32 patients to include Marsh scores 0 through 3 and reported a lower specificity of 63.6% comparing VCE findings and histology. They recommended that when VCE, done for any reason, detects villus atrophy, a biopsy should follow because the correlation with abnormal histology is high. However, a normal VCE does not exclude villus atrophy. This condition is also true for endoscopy; the absence of optical endoscopic features of celiac disease does not exclude celiac disease, and random biopsy of normal appearing mucosa is recommended.[21]

Interobserver agreement varies in studies based on the experience of the VCE reader. The interpretation of studies is subjective and agreement may be poor among capsule readers with limited exposure to celiac disease. Petroniene and colleagues[16] found the sensitivity and specificity of the test was 100% with experienced VCE readers, but agreement was poor among inexperienced readers. Rondonotti and colleagues[18] showed agreement ranging from 79.2% to 94.4% with kappa values indicating moderate to excellent agreement. Biagi and colleagues[20] proposed a 3-grade scale to standardize mucosal atrophy reading, but noted high interobserver variability, again suggesting that experience in VCE interpretation is important. With more experience in VCE reading and adoption of structured terminology of capsule findings, improvement in reader agreement is expected.[22,23]

In a recent multicenter, retrospective study,[24] 163 patients with suspicion of celiac disease who underwent VCE were analyzed for diagnostic yield, therapeutic impact, and safety. The diagnostic yield for all patients was 54% to include villus atrophy, complicated celiac disease, and other enteropathies. VCE results changed the therapeutic approach in 71.8% of cases. In patients with positive serology and negative atrophy on biopsy, VCE found intestinal atrophy in more than one-half of this group of 39 patients. These patients were treated with a gluten-free diet and 66.7% responded. They concluded that VCE was valuable in this group and that villus atrophy was missed owing to patchy distribution that may be more distal and not reached by endoscopic biopsies.

DOES VIDEO CAPSULE ENDOSCOPY HAVE A ROLE IN MONITORING?

One potential new application for VCE is noninvasive evaluation of the response to a gluten-free diet. Murray and colleagues[3] performed VCE on 35 patients at the time of celiac disease diagnosis, confirmed with duodenal biopsy and serology. VCE identified the distribution of villus atrophy; 59% showed extensive enteropathy from duodenum into the jejunum, 32% had villus changes confined to the duodenum, and 1 patient had villus changes seen only in the jejunum. Follow-up VCE showed that after a gluten-free diet for more than 6 months, healing occurred from distal to proximal in the small bowel.

Lidum and colleagues[25] evaluated the symptoms, serology, duodenal biopsy, and VCE in 12 patients after 1 year on a gluten-free diet. They also found healing from distal to proximal. Importantly, in some patients duodenal follow-up biopsy remained abnormal, although their symptom scores, serology, and extent of villus atrophy on capsule examination improved. They concluded that small bowel mucosal healing as determined by VCE correlates with improvement in symptoms and that duodenal biopsy does not show the extent of improvement that has occurred more distally.

The European Society of Gastrointestinal Endoscopy guidelines[12] state that, at the present time, there is no role for the use of VCE to evaluate the extent of disease or response to a gluten free diet. More studies are needed to demonstrate a relationship between the quantitative extent of disease and severity of clinical presentation (**Boxes 1** and **2**).

CAPSULE ENDOSCOPY IN REFRACTORY CELIAC DISEASE

Capsule endoscopy has been evaluated in nonresponsive and refractory celiac disease. Patients with refractory celiac disease, particularly type II, are at risk for developing complications such as intestinal T-cell lymphoma and ulcerative jejunitis. These lesions are more commonly seen in the more distal small bowel[26–28] (**Fig. 3**).

Barret and colleagues[29] looked at the diagnostic yield of VCE in refractory celiac disease in 9 patients with symptomatic celiac disease, 11 patients with refractory celiac disease type I, and 18 patients with refractory celiac disease type II, and 45 patients without celiac disease. Villus atrophy and distal ulcers were more common in patients with celiac disease than controls. Low serum albumin correlated with more extensive mucosal disease and refractory celiac disease type II. Lymphoma was found in 3 patients.

In a study by Daum and colleagues,[27] 7 patients with refractory celiac disease type I and 7 patients with refractory celiac disease type II were examined by VCE, upper and lower endoscopy, and imaging with an abdominal computed tomography scan or MR tomography. Two patients had findings of intestinal T-cell lymphoma or jejunitis and 1 was found only by VCE. The other case was diagnosed by lymphadenopathy seen on computed tomography/MR tomography. This confirmed the value of VCE as well as other imaging modalities in patients with refractory celiac disease type II. They found no diagnostic benefit with advanced imaging in refractory celiac disease type I.

Other studies have frequently found positive celiac serologies in patients with nonresponsive celiac disease after adhering to a gluten-free diet for at least 6 months.[28] This finding supports eliminating other factors that can cause persistent symptoms before proceeding with further evaluation with VCE. Inadvertent gluten

---

Box 1
Recommendations for VCE in celiac disease

1. Strong recommendation against VCE to make an initial diagnosis of celiac disease except for suspected celiac disease in a patient who is unable or unwilling to have a conventional endoscopy.

2. Equivocal diagnosis. Positive celiac serology but normal small bowel biopsy[11,12] (not all guidelines supportive[13]).

3. Celiac disease with unexplained or alarm symptoms, refractory celiac disease especially type II. Strong recommendation.

4. Currently no role for VCE in evaluating the extent of disease or response to a gluten free diet. Further studies needed.[12]

Abbreviation: VCE, video capsule endoscopy.

Box 2
Video capsule endoscopy in celiac disease: limitations to use

1. Unable to biopsy for tissue diagnosis.

2. Partial villus atrophy may be difficult to identify.

3. Interpretation is subjective and requires experience

4. There is interobserver variability.

5. Studies maybe incomplete

6. Possible additional cost factors.

---

ingestion is common and can occur in up to 50% of patients. Others causes of continuing symptoms include lactose intolerance, fructose intolerance, small intestinal bacterial overgrowth, pancreatic insufficiency, irritable bowel syndrome, and microscopic colitis.[30]

The study by Atlas and colleagues[28] also found ulcerations and erosions of the small bowel in 18% of nonresponsive patients with celiac disease, 19% of controls, and 33% of uncomplicated celiac disease, and associated this with aspirin and nonsteroidal antiinflammatory drug use. They also identified 1 adenocarcinoma and 1 ulcerative jejunitis complication.

Efthymakis and colleagues[31] studied 26 patients with celiac disease and persistent iron deficiency anemia after at least 24 months on a gluten-free diet with documentation of normal celiac serologies. Iron deficiency anemia is a common finding at diagnosis and usually resolves after 12 months on a gluten-free diet.[32] Patients had an esophogastroduodenoscopy, colonoscopy, and VCE. VCE found significant disease in 3 patients including erosive jejunitis, and on subsequent enteroscopy and biopsy one was diagnosed as having refractory celiac disease type II and two were diagnosed as having Crohn's disease. They found a low albumin to be associated with the presence of more mucosal pathology, as was also seen in the study by Barret and colleagues[29]

VCE has identified complications of celiac disease such as lymphomas, adenocarcinomas, and ulcerative ileojejunitis, as well as other conditions such as Crohn's disease.[26–29] In a large, retrospective, multicenter European study,[33] 189 patients with

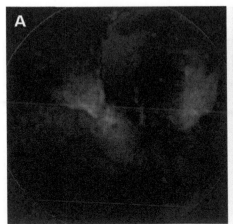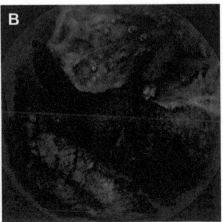

Fig. 3. (A) jejunal adenocarcinoma in celiac disease. (B) Ulcerative jejunitis.

celiac disease had VCE for nonresponsive celiac disease (n = 103), or celiac disease with alarm symptoms (n = 86). Findings included atrophic mucosa (48.7%), ulcerative jejunoileitis (11.1%), intestinal lymphoma (3.7%), and other enteropathies (3.7% including Crohn's disease and 1 neuroendocrine tumor). The overall diagnostic yield was 67.2% and this modified management in 59.3% of cases. They found the diagnostic yield was higher in the nonresponsive celiac disease group. They note that VCE had to be combined with other modalities such as balloon-assisted enteroscopy for histologic diagnosis. VCE was found to be valuable in the management of complicated celiac disease to identify or exclude significant pathology and guide deep enteroscopy.

Multiple guidelines recommend VCE in patients with celiac disease with unexplained persistent symptoms despite a gluten-free diet.

CAPSULE ENDOSCOPY AND CELIAC DISEASE: FUTURE DEVELOPMENTS

Limitations in the use of capsule endoscopy in celiac disease include subjective interpretation, its labor intensive nature, and an inability to detect mild villus atrophy. Virtual chromoendoscopy has been incorporated into capsule endoscopy. Flexible spectral imaging color enhancement, and blue mode filtering have been looked at to evaluate the usefulness of this technology primarily for increasing detection of vascular lesions and ulcerations.[34] The use of the 3 flexible spectral imaging color enhancement modes has not been shown to improve the detection rate for angioectasias and ulcers in a recent metaanalysis.[35] This visualization strategy has not been applied to capsule endoscopy and celiac disease.

There is much interest in the development of an observer-independent diagnostic method that could potentially bypass the difficulties in interpretation of both biopsy and capsule endoscopy for celiac disease. The development of an automated system for predicting celiac disease is being investigated.[36] Such technology could save costs, time, and manpower, and possibly increase safety if in some cases biopsies could ultimately be avoided.[37]

Ciaccio and colleagues[38] have reported on a computer-assisted method to detect and quantify villus atrophy by capsule endoscopy. Computer analysis of the 2-dimensional capsule image is used to generate a 3-dimensional mucosal structure, using shape-from-shading principles to measure the villus protrusions and detect and quantify villus atrophy. As compared with controls, patients with celiac disease and villus atrophy have more blunted protrusions. Image analysis is also done for texture differences between patients with celiac disease and controls. In VCE images of patients with celiac disease, there is significantly greater texture, which is a measure of the degree of variance in the images. Microscopic villus atrophy and macroscopic scalloping of folds, fissures, and mosaic pattern increase the heterogeneity of the pixel gray scale. The structural variation in patients with celiac disease with villus atrophy results in increased measure of texture. Quantitative image analysis has also been used to estimate motility by evaluating dynamic properties in a sequence of images and also by using the frequency spectrum generated by a series of capsule images. Using these methods and a polling protocol, villus atrophy was predicted with a sensitivity of 83.9% and specificity of 92.9%.[36] Further studies are now being done to validate this system in a larger study population.[38]

Summary

The role of capsule endoscopy in the diagnosis and monitoring of celiac disease is still being determined. Current consensus opinion limits VCE for diagnostic use under special circumstances, such as patients who are unwilling or medically unable to have an upper endoscopy. There are strong recommendations against using VCE to make an initial diagnosis owing to its lower sensitivity to detect partial villus atrophy[13,39] and the need for duodenal biopsy for diagnosis in such patients. Positive celiac serology (tissue transglutaminase or EMA) and normal duodenal histology is a potential indication for VCE, although it is not supported by all studies.[18,25,40] In addition, a study by Kurien and colleagues[41] supports the use of VCE in equivocal cases of celiac disease with negative serology and villus atrophy or Marsh 1 and 2 lesions with a diagnostic yield of 18%. This and future study results may prompt change to the recommendations in those with equivocal celiac disease.

VCE is indicated in patients with celiac disease with alarm symptoms and particularly refractory celiac disease type II. VCE is only part of the evaluation, which includes upper endoscopy, colonoscopy, radiographic enterography, and device-assisted enteroscopy. The main limitation of VCE is the inability to obtain biopsies. Villus atrophy is not specific for celiac diagnosis. VCE interpretation is also subjective and dependent on the experience of the capsule reader. There is a risk of capsule retention in patients with refractory celiac disease type II and obstructive symptoms owing to stenosis related to ulcerative jejunitis, lymphoma, or in adenocarcinoma.

ENTEROSCOPY IN CELIAC DISEASE

Celiac disease involves predominantly the proximal small bowel, the first site of gluten exposure. In most patients, inflammation is found in the duodenum, which is easily reachable by standard endoscopy for diagnosis. Rarely, celiac disease spares the duodenum and involves the jejunum alone.[42] In such patients, enteroscopy is required for diagnosis. In a prospective study of push enteroscopy in responsive and refractory celiac disease, Cellier and colleagues[43] found similar endoscopic and histologic findings in the duodenum and jejunum of responsive celiac disease. Four patients had villus atrophy that was more severe in the duodenum than jejunum but this finding did not change management. Although there is little role for enteroscopy in the diagnosis of celiac disease, it is very useful to evaluate complications of the disease.

Celiac disease is associated with an increased risk for GI cancers that include adenocarcinoma of the small bowel (**Fig. 4**).

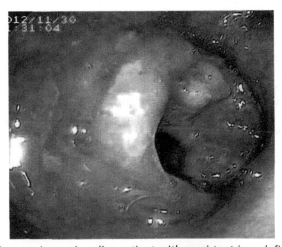

Fig. 4. Jejunal adenocarcinoma in celiac patient with persistent iron deficiency anemia.

Rarely (0.31%),[44] patients with celiac disease fail to respond to a gluten-free diet exhibit alarm symptoms and are diagnosed with refractory celiac disease. A subset of these patients, have aberrant intraepithelial T cells (refractory celiac disease type II) and develop ulcerative jejunitis and enteropathy-associated T-cell lymphoma (EATL) that is associated with a poor 5-year survival.[45] Patients with refractory celiac disease are usually older, male, and have severe diarrhea, weight loss, and hypoproteinemia. Occasionally, obstructive symptoms are present owing to small bowel ulceration and stenosis. Duodenal biopsies in refractory disease show severe villus atrophy, but ulcerating lesions and lymphoma are often deep in the small bowel, out of reach of standard endoscopy and require enteroscopy for diagnosis and management (Box 3).

THE ROLE OF DEVICE-ASSIST ENTEROSCOPY IN CELIAC DISEASE

In 2001, Yamamoto[46] developed an enteroscope and overtube device with balloons at both ends to allow pleating of bowel on the back of the overtube and advancement of the enteroscope deep into the small bowel using a push and pull technique. Since then, other devices have become available for deep enteroscopy: single-balloon enteroscopy that uses a single balloon on the tip of the over tube, spiral enteroscopy that uses an overtube with spiral ridges and rotational energy to pleat bowel for advancement, and a through-the-scope balloon device using standard endoscopy.[47] These techniques are labor intensive, have steep learning curves and require dedicated staff. In small studies, the devices have similar diagnostic yields. Complications include bowel perforation, bleeding, and pancreatitis.[47] device-assist enteroscopy has revolutionized the diagnosis and therapy of small bowel disease, particularly small bowel bleeding and tumors.

The use of device-assist enteroscopy in celiac disease remains limited owing to the rare nature of the type of this complicated disease. Studies are few, small, and predominately used double-balloon enteroscopy (DBE). In a study of patients with refractory celiac disease by Hadithi and colleagues,[48] EATL was found in 5 of 21 patients (24%) and ulcerative jejunitis in 2 of 21 patients (9%). Endoscopic appearances of EATL included circumferential, discrete, or confluent ulcerations. In 4 patients with computed tomography findings suggestive of small bowel wall thickening, EATL was excluded. DBE was useful to both diagnose and exclude EATL. Tomba and colleagues[49] reported on VCE and DBE in 53 patients with poor response or nonadherence to a gluten-free diet and alarm symptoms. DBE detected 3 malignancies (5.7%), 2 jejunal adenocarcinomas, and 1 ileal neuroendocrine tumor.

In a recent metaanalysis by Elli and colleagues[50] on the use of VCE and enteroscopy to detect malignant and premalignant small bowel lesions in 515 patients with complicated celiac disease, only 3 European studies (76 patients) met inclusion criteria using push enteroscopy or DBE. There were 8 small bowel malignancies (10%) detected—5 EATL, 2 adenocarcinoma, and 1 neuroendocrine tumor. Ulcerative jejunitis was found in 13 patients (17%). The overall diagnostic yield for enteroscopy was 27%. VCE and

---

Box 3
Recommendations for enteroscopy in celiac disease

1. Strong clinical suspicion of celiac disease with negative duodenal biopsies[42] or equivocal diagnosis.

2. Celiac disease with unexplained or alarm symptoms, suspected malignancy, and refractory celiac disease especially type II.[48–50]

enteroscopy were effective to detect small bowel malignancies and ulcerative jejunitis in complicated celiac disease.

SUMMARY

VCE is more sensitive than standard endoscopy to detect villus atrophy and define the extent of disease with good interobserver agreement with experienced capsule readers; however, it lacks the capacity to take a biopsy. VCE is currently used to assist in the diagnosis of celiac disease in special circumstances when duodenal biopsy is not possible. The role of VCE in the diagnosis and monitoring of celiac disease is evolving. Computer-assisted diagnosis by analysis of villus changes and motility using quantitative image analysis will be helpful in the future usefulness of VCE in celiac disease.

VCE and enteroscopy combined with radiographic enterography have proven benefit in patients with complicated celiac disease (alarm symptoms, iron deficiency anemia, refractory celiac disease type II, and suspected ulcerative jejunitis, T-cell lymphoma, or small bowel adenocarcinoma). Advances in VCE and device-assist enteroscopy design with developments enabling capsule biopsy and locomotion[51] and a motorized spiral device for enteroscopy are in development.

REFERENCES

1. Van de Bruaene C, De Looze D, Hindryckx P. Small bowel capsule endoscopy: where are we after almost 15 years of use? World J Gastrointest Endosc 2015; 7(1):13–36.
2. Green PH, Cellier C. Celiac disease. N Engl J Med 2007;357:1731–43.
3. Murray JA, Rubio-Tapia A, van Dyke CT, et al. Mucosal atrophy in celiac disease: extent of involvement, correlation with clinical presentation, and response to treatment. Clin Gastroenterol Hepatol 2008;6(2):186–93.
4. Horoldt BS, McAlindon ME, Stephenson TJ, et al. Making the diagnosis of celiac disease: is there a role for push enteroscopy? Eur J Gastroenterol Hepatol 2004; 16:1143–6.
5. Ravelli A, Bolognini S, Gambarotti M, et al. Variability of histologic lesions in relation to biopsy site in gluten-sensitive enteropathy. Am J Gastroenterol 2005;100: 177–85.
6. Kav T, Sokmensuer C, Sivri B. Enteroscopic findings of celiac disease and their correlation with mucosal histopathologic changes. Comput Biol Med 2015;65: 315–9.
7. Lebwohl B, Kapel RC, Neugut A, et al. Adherence to biopsy guidelines increases celiac disease diagnosis. Gastrointest Endosc 2011;74:103–9.
8. Arguelles-Grande C, Tennyson CA, Lewis SK, et al. Variability in small bowel histopathology reporting between different pathology practice settings: impact on the diagnosis of celiac disease. J Clin Pathol 2012;63:242–7.
9. Soncini M, Girelli CM, de Franchis R, et al, SBCE Lombardia Study Group; On behalf AIGO, SIED and SIGE Lombardia. Small-bowel capsule endoscopy in clinical practice: has anything changed over 13 years? Dig Dis Sci 2018. https://doi.org/10.1007/s10620-018-5101-9.
10. Petroniene R, Dubcenco E, Baker JP, et al. Given capsule endoscopy in celiac disease. Gastrointest Endosc Clin N Am 2004;14:115–27.
11. Cellier C, Green PH, Collin P, et al. ICCE consensus for celiac disease. Endoscopy 2005;37:1055–9.

12. Pennazio M, Spada C, Eliakim R, et al. Small-bowel capsule endoscopy and device-assisted enteroscopy for diagnosis and treatment of small-bowel disorders: European Society of Gastrointestinal Endoscopy (ESGE) clinical guideline. Endoscopy 2015;47(4):352–76.
13. Enns RA, Hookey L, Armstrong D, et al. Clinical practice guidelines for the use of video capsule endoscopy. Gastroenterology 2017;152(3):497–514.
14. Brocchi E, Tomassetti P, Misitano B, et al. Endoscopic markers in adult coeliac disease. Dig Liver Dis 2002;34(3):177–82.
15. Tursi A, Brandimarte G, Giorgetti GM, et al. Endoscopic features of celiac disease in adults and their correlation with age, histological damage, and clinical form of the disease. Endoscopy 2002;34:787–92.
16. Petroniene R, Dubcenco E, Baker JP, et al. Given capsule endoscopy in celiac disease: evaluation of diagnostic accuracy and interobserver agreement. Am J Gastroenterol 2005;100:685–94.
17. Spada C, Riccioni ME, Urgesi R, et al. Capsule endoscopy in celiac disease. World J Gastroenterol 2008;14(26):4146–51.
18. Rondonotti E, Spada C, Cave D, et al. Video capsule enteroscopy in the diagnosis of celiac disease: a multicenter study. Am J Gastroenterol 2007;102:1624–31.
19. Rokkas T, Niv Y. The role of video capsule endoscopy in the diagnosis of celiac disease: a meta-analysis. Eur J Gastroenterol Hepatol 2012;24:303–8.
20. Biagi F, Rondonotti E, Campanella J, et al. Video capsule endoscopy and histology for small-bowel mucosa evaluation: a comparison performed by blinded observers. Clin Gastroenterol Hepatol 2006;4:998–1003.
21. Lee SK, Green PH. Endoscopy in celiac disease. Curr Opin Gastroenterol 2005; 21(5):589–94.
22. Jang BI, Lee SH, Moon JS, et al. Inter-observer agreement on the interpretation of capsule endoscopy findings based on capsule endoscopy structured terminology: a multicenter study by the Korean Gut Image Study Group. Scand J Gastroenterol 2010;45(3):370–4.
23. Korman LY, Delvaux M, Gay G, et al. Capsule endoscopy structured terminology (CEST): proposal of a standardized and structured terminology for reporting capsule endoscopy procedures [review]. Endoscopy 2005;37(10):951–9.
24. Luján-Sanchis M, Pérez-Cuadrado-Robles E, García-Lledó J, et al. Role of capsule endoscopy in suspected celiac disease: a European multi-centre study. World J Gastroenterol 2017;23(4):703–11.
25. Lidums I, Teo E, Field J, et al. Capsule endoscopy: a valuable tool in the follow-up of people with celiac disease on a gluten-free diet. Clin Transl Gastroenterol 2011;2:e4.
26. Cuilliford A, Daly J, Diamond B, et al. The value of wireless capsule endoscopy in patients with complicated celiac disease. Gastrointest Endosc 2005;62:55–61.
27. Daum S, Wahnschaffe U, Glasenapp R, et al. Capsule endoscopy in refractory celiac disease. Endoscopy 2007;39(5):455–8.
28. Atlas DS, Rubio-Tapia A, Van Dyke CT, et al. Capsule endoscopy in nonresponsive celiac disease. Gastrointest Endosc 2011;74(6):1315–22.
29. Barret M, Malamut G, Rahmi G, et al. Diagnostic yield of capsule endoscopy in refractory celiac disease. Am J Gastroenterol 2012;107(10):1546–53.
30. Abdulkarim AS, Burgart LJ, See J, et al. Etiology of nonresponsive celiac disease: results of a systematic approach. Am J Gastroenterol 2002;97(8):2016–21.
31. Efthymakis K, Milano A, Laterza F, et al. Iron deficiency anemia despite effective gluten-free diet in celiac disease: diagnostic role of small bowel capsule endoscopy. Dig Liver Dis 2017;49(4):412–6.

32. Annibale B, Severi C, Christolini A, et al. Efficacy of gluten-free diet alone on recovery from iron deficiency anemia in adult celiac patients. Am J Gastroenterol 2001;96(1):132–7.
33. Perez-Cuadrado-Robles E, Lujan-Sanchis M, Elli L, et al. Role of capsule endoscopy in alarm features and non-responsive celiac disease: a European multicenter study. Dig Endosc 2017. https://doi.org/10.1111/den.13002.
34. Negreanu L, Preda CM, Ionescu D, et al. Progress in digestive endoscopy: flexible spectral imaging colour enhancement (FICE)- technical review. J Med Life 2015;8(4):416–22.
35. Yung DE, Boal Carvalho P, Giannakou A, et al. Clinical validity of flexible spectral imaging color enhancement (FICE) in small-bowel capsule endoscopy: a systematic review and meta-analysis. Endoscopy 2017;49(3):258–69.
36. Ciaccio EJ, Tennyson CA, Bhagat G, et al. Implementation of a polling protocol for predicting celiac disease in videocapsule analysis. World J Gastrointest Endosc 2013;5:313–22.
37. Hegenbart S, Uhl A, Vecsei A. Survey on computer aided decision support for diagnosis of celiac disease. Comput Biol Med 2015;65:348–58.
38. Ciaccio EJ, Lewis SK, Bhagat G, et al. Coeliac disease and the videocapsule: what have we learned till now. Ann Transl Med 2017;5:197.
39. Delvaux M, Gay G. International conference on capsule and double- balloon endoscopy (ICCD) Paris,27-28 August 2010. Endoscopy 2011;43(6):533–9.
40. Chang MS, Rubin M, Lewis SK, et al. Diagnosing celiac disease by video capsule endoscopy (VCE) when esophogastroduodenoscopy (EGD) and biopsy is unable to provide a diagnosis: a case series. BMC Gastroenterol 2012;12:90.
41. Kurien M, Evans KE, Aziz I, et al. Capsule endoscopy in adult celiac disease: a potential role in equivocal cases of celiac disease? Gastrointest Endosc 2013;77:227–32.
42. Valitutti F, Di Nardo G, Barbato M, et al. Mapping histologic patchiness of celiac disease by push enteroscopy. Gastrointest Endosc 2014;79:95–100.
43. Cellier C, Cuillerier E, Patey-Mariaud de Serre N, et al. Push enteroscopy in celiac sprue and refractory sprue. Gastrointest Endosc 1999;50:613–7.
44. Ilus T, Kaukinen K, Virta LJ, et al. Refractory coeliac disease in a country with a high prevalence of clinically-diagnosed coeliac disease. Aliment Pharmacol Ther 2014;39:418–25.
45. Cellier C, Delabesse E, Helmer C, et al. Refractory sprue, coeliac disease, and enteropathy-associated T-cell lymphoma. Lancet 2000;356:203–8.
46. Yamamoto H, Sekine Y, Sato Y, et al. Total enteroscopy with a nonsurgical steerable double-balloon method. Gastrointest Endosc 2001;53:216–20.
47. Micic D, Semrad CE. Small bowel endoscopy. Curr Treat Options Gastroenterol 2016;14:220–35.
48. Hadithi M, Al-toma A, Oudejans J, et al. The value of double-balloon enteroscopy in patients with refractory celiac disease. Am J Gastroenterol 2007;102:987–96.
49. Tomba C, Elli L, Bardella MT, et al. Enteroscopy for the early detection of small bowel tumours in at-risk celiac patients. Dig Liver Dis 2014;46:400–4.
50. Elli L, Casazza G, Locatelli M, et al. Use of enteroscopy for the detection of malignant and premalignant lesions of the small bowel in complicated celiac disease: a meta-analysis. Gastrointest Endosc 2017;86(2):264–73.e1.
51. Cuiti G, Caliò R, Camboni D, et al. Frontiers of robotic endoscopic capsules: a review. J Microbio Robot 2016;11(1):1–18.

(Outcome) Measure for (Intervention) Measures

A Guide to Choosing the Appropriate Noninvasive Clinical Outcome Measure for Intervention Studies in Celiac Disease

Prashant Singh, MB BS[a], Jocelyn A. Silvester, MD, PhD[b,c],*,
Daniel Leffler, MD, MS[a,d]

KEYWORDS

- Celiac disease • Intervention studies • Outcome measures • Study design
- Patient-reported outcomes

KEY POINTS

- There is an unmet need for dietary and behavioral interventions for celiac disease.
- The existence of a dietary approach to celiac disease management complicates selection of outcome measures.
- Serology and histology are more likely to be appropriate as safety outcomes rather than primary outcomes.
- The available patient-reported outcomes for celiac disease have significant limitations.
- The burden of disease is more appropriate for real-world studies than for clinical trials.

Disclosure Statement: J.A. Silvester has served on advisory boards for Takeda Pharmaceuticals Inc and is supported by a National Institutes of Health T32 training grant (DK 07760). D. Leffler serves as a medical director and receives a salary from Takeda Pharmaceuticals. P. Singh received salary support from NIH T32 DK 07760.
[a] Harvard Celiac Disease Research Program, Department of Medicine, Division of Gastroenterology, Beth Israel Deaconess Medical Center, 330 Brookline Avenue, Boston, MA 02215, USA; [b] Harvard Celiac Disease Research Program, Beth Israel Deaconess Medical Center, 330 Brookline Avenue, Boston, MA 02215, USA; [c] Division of Gastroenterology and Nutrition, Boston Children's Hospital, 300 Longwood Avenue, Boston, MA 02215, USA; [d] Gastroenterology Therapeutic Area Research and Development, Takeda Pharmaceuticals, 40 Landsdowne Street, Boston, MA 02139, USA
* Corresponding author. Boston Children's Hospital, Hunnewell Ground, 300 Longwood Avenue, Boston, MA 02115.
E-mail address: jsilves2@bidmc.harvard.edu

Gastroenterol Clin N Am 48 (2019) 85–99
https://doi.org/10.1016/j.gtc.2018.09.006
0889-8553/19/© 2018 Elsevier Inc. All rights reserved.

INTRODUCTION

Lifelong strict adherence to a gluten-free diet (GFD) has been the primary treatment of celiac disease (CD) for nearly a century and has remained so even as understanding of the disease has increased.[1,2] Despite availability of accurate and available diagnostic tests, most individuals with CD remain undiagnosed, suggesting there is a need for enhanced screening strategies. Although diagnosis is a major hurdle in CD treatment, problems can persist after therapy is instituted. An imperfect treatment, the GFD is practically, psychologically, and financially challenging with a patient-reported treatment burden comparable with that of end-stage renal disease.[3] In addition, restrictive diets, including a GFD, are more likely to be nutritionally imbalanced.[4] Even more problematic, up to 30% of patients with CD on a GFD have ongoing symptoms and/or persistent villus atrophy.[5] For these reasons, dietary and behavioral interventions are needed to improve outcomes for the millions of patients trying to follow a GFD. Despite the relative lack of progress to date, the discovery pipeline is starting to flow with vaccines and other pharmacologic interventions currently in development, some of which have already been tested in phase 1 and 2 clinical trials and require thoughtful study to assess their impact on symptoms, disease outcomes, and quality of life.

Generally, interventional CD studies are grouped into two main categories: real-world trials and clinical trials. Real-world trials usually involve either diagnosis or behavioral and dietary approaches to improve dietary adherence, diet quality, and/or quality of life on a GFD. Real-world trials involve pragmatic changes that patients implement in real-life settings, thus allowing for evaluation of the impact of treatment on quality of life, social function, and related end points, which are not feasible in the setting of most randomized clinical trials. Conversely, clinical trials are performed in controlled settings often for assessment of novel biomarkers, pharmacologic adjuncts to a GFD, or pharmacologic alternatives to a GFD that allow for unrestricted gluten ingestion. In clinical trials, objectives and time frames are discrete and well-defined allowing for use of specific targeted outcomes, such as patient-reported outcomes (PRO) measured symptoms or intestinal histology, as discussed later. Clinical trials are time efficient for assessment of the effects of interventions on these outcomes but, by definition, are only approximations of the real-life experiences of patients with any given disorder. This is especially true in CD with its complex intersection of long-term complications; acute and chronic symptoms; and the social, economic, and nutritional consequences of the current treatment, a GFD (**Fig. 1**). For these reasons, assessing the overall human impact of interventions, whether of diagnosis, support, or treatment, in CD requires real-world studies.

Selecting appropriate end points for intervention studies in CD is especially important given the large number of patients who may potentially benefit. Biopsy-confirmed CD has a pooled global prevalence of 0.7%,[6] which is greater than the prevalence of Crohn's disease and ulcerative colitis combined. The existence of a dietary approach to management of CD complicates selection of outcome measures. Particularly for pharmacologic adjuncts and alternatives to a GFD, gluten exposure must be assessed and considered in the analysis, yet it may not be a meaningful measure of the efficacy of the intervention being studied.

Small intestinal histology and serology are essential outcomes to include in assessment of novel treatment interventions for CD, but in many cases may not be appropriate primary end points. Practical limitations of histology as a primary outcome in CD include invasiveness, interobserver variability in interpretation, sampling error caused by the patchy nature of the celiac mucosal lesion, and lack of ability to assess

Celiac Disease Outcomes of Interest

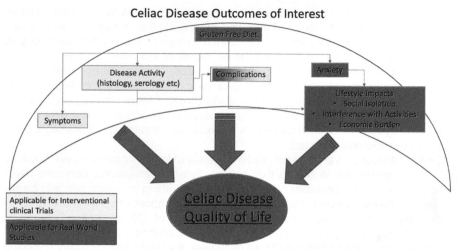

Fig. 1. Conceptual model of celiac disease outcome measures for clinical trials and real-world settings. Many factors influence quality of life in celiac disease. Some (*yellow shading*) are more appropriate for real-world setting, whereas others (*shaded gray*) are more applicable in clinical trial settings.

extent of intestinal disease.[7] These limitations likely contribute to the inconsistent association between histologic findings and some long-term outcomes,[8–10] and observed variability in kinetics of mucosal damage. Although more practical to obtain, serum levels of antibodies directed to tissue transglutaminase or (deamidated) gliadin do not correlate closely with histologic damage in patients with CD on a GFD[11] nor are they responsive to gluten challenge.[12] It is possible that a drug that ameliorates symptoms may actually lead to worsening in histology or serology by allowing for greater gluten exposure. The currently available treatment of CD (ie, GFD) has few serious direct adverse effects, so the safety profile for any new therapy intended as an adjunct to or replacement of a GFD must be extremely favorable. Thus, the appropriate role of serology and histology in clinical trials may be as important safety outcomes rather than a primary outcome.

Consistent with this paradigm, the third Gastroenterology Regulatory Endpoints and Advancement of Therapeutics workshop, which was sponsored by the Food and Drug Administration (FDA), recommended that PROs seem to be most suitable as primary outcomes in phase 2 and 3 clinical trials for CD either as sole end point or as coprimary end point with other objective measures.[13] Although health-related quality of life (HRQoL) might be a more relevant concern for patients with CD compared with individual symptoms, it might be less amenable to change with therapeutic interventions. Given the multidimensional nature of HRQoL, certain aspects of HRQoL might be nonmodifiable or might be confounded by factors unrelated to CD.

In this article, we review noninvasive clinical outcome measures and provide case scenarios to illustrate key considerations in selecting appropriate clinical outcome measures for treatment interventions in CD.

MEASURES OF INTESTINAL FUNCTION AND NUTRITION

CD causes impaired intestinal absorptive function, particularly in the duodenum. Classical measures of intestinal permeability, such as lactulose-mannitol fractional excretion, are difficult to administer and have had mixed results, with significant inter-individual variability that may be of a greater magnitude than intraindividual changes observed during gluten challenge.[12] In contrast, serum levels of intestinal fatty acid binding protein, a proposed marker of small intestinal epithelial damage, are more sensitive to gluten challenge[14] and to a GFD.[15] Despite responsiveness within individuals, absolute levels of intestinal fatty acid binding protein do not correlate well with histologic damage in the population, even at diagnosis.[15] More recently, oral bioavailability of simvastatin, which is primarily metabolized by cytochrome P450 3A4 in villus type enterocytes, has been proposed as a functional measure of villus integrity, but has not been thoroughly tested.[16]

Nutritional measures are an even cruder measure of intestinal function, yet they may play a role, particularly in studies that involve dietary interventions. Clinically, treatment of villus atrophy increases nutrient absorption leading to weight gain and development of metabolic syndrome,[17] both of which are important considerations given many patients are already overweight at the time of CD diagnosis.[18,19] Iron is absorbed from villus tips in the proximal duodenum, so it may be especially relevant as a marker of malabsorption in CD. At diagnosis, iron deficiency is highly prevalent and anemia may be a marker of disease severity.[20] Malabsorption of other nutrients, such as zinc, vitamin B_{12}, or folate, is less common at diagnosis, but may reflect more extensive enteropathy or may develop on a GFD.[4]

PATIENT-REPORTED OUTCOMES FOR MEASUREMENT OF CELIAC DISEASE SYMPTOMS

The FDA recommends that PROs should meet the following criteria: content validity (extent to which instrument measures the concept/domain it is used to measure), construct validity (evidence that instrument correlates with another accepted measure of disease activity), criterion validity (degree to which instrument is a reflection of an accepted gold standard), test-retest reliability, and responsiveness to change.[21] However, there are several challenges when using PROs in CD. This includes determining an appropriate gold standard to determine criterion validity. There is no clear relationship between histology and CD symptoms, which range from classic gastrointestinal symptoms, such as abdominal pain and diarrhea, to nongastrointestinal symptoms, such as ataxia, headache, and infertility.[2] In addition, a small yet important proportion of patients who are diagnosed by screening of high-risk groups, such as first-degree relatives, type 1 diabetes may be completely asymptomatic.[2] This is different from other chronic gastrointestinal diseases, such as inflammatory bowel disease, in which most patients present with gastrointestinal symptoms alone and there is a closer correlation between intestinal damage and symptoms.[22]

Significant symptom heterogeneity associated with CD makes it difficult to have a single PRO, which would be appropriate for all patients with celiac. It also makes studying responsiveness to change in CD a challenging task. In addition, studies have shown that symptom severity in CD does not correlate well with objective measures of disease activity (off and on treatment), an observation that is not unique to CD. Despite these challenges with PRO development in CD, there has been progress in the last few years, and a summary of available PROs in CD is given later.

Gastrointestinal symptoms are a main concern and reason for clinical evaluation for patients with CD, thus most PROs focus predominantly on gastrointestinal symptoms (**Table 1**). Although generic PRO, such as the Gastrointestinal Symptom Rating Scale (GSRS), are not specific for CD, they have been shown to correlate with established markers of CD activity, such as histology, at diagnosis.[23] In addition, they have also

Table 1
Commonly used patient-reported outcome measures for celiac disease interventional studies

	Format	Domains	Recall Period	Regulatory End Point[a]	Comments
Symptom Measure					
Generic					
GSRS[25]	15 items, each rated on intensity, frequency, duration, and impact of daily living with (7-point scale)	• Abdominal pain • Diarrhea • Constipation • Reflux • Indigestion	Preceding month	No	• Correlates with histology at diagnosis[23] • Population norms available • Interview or self-report • Modified CD-GSRS
CD specific					
Celiac Symptom Index[26]	16 items, 5-point Likert scale	• Intestinal symptoms • Extraintestinal symptoms • General health	Past 4 wk	No	• Most extensively studied CD-specific PRO
Celiac Disease PRO[24]	11 items, Visual Analogue Scale from no discomfort (0) to worst possible discomfort (10)	• Intestinal symptoms • Extraintestinal symptoms	1 d	Yes	• Construct validity and responsiveness to change not reported
Celiac Disease Symptom Diary[29]	10 symptoms, scaled 0–10	• Intestinal symptoms • Extraintestinal symptoms • Value in health paper	Each symptom assessed daily on 0–10 scale over 7 d to give an overall score of 0–70	Yes	• Construct validity and responsiveness to change not reported

(continued on next page)

Table 1
(continued)

	Format	Domains	Recall Period	Regulatory End Point[a]	Comments
Quality of Life Measures					
Generic					

SF-36[30]	36 items, various scales	• Physical health
		  ○ Functioning
		  ○ Role
		  ○ Bodily pain
		  ○ General health
		• Mental health
		  ○ Vitality
		  ○ Social
		  ○ Emotional
		  ○ Mental health
			Past 4 wk	No	• Population norms available for healthy and other diseases
					• Gold standard for quality of life scale development

PGWBI[31]	22 items, 6-point Likert scale	• Vitality • General Health • Self-control • Anxiety • Positive well-being • Depressed mood	Past month	No	• Does not address physiologic function or vitality
CD specific					
Celiac Disease Quality of Life Survey[32]	20 items, 5-point Likert scale	• Dysphoria • Inadequate treatment • Limitations • Health concerns	Past month (30 d)	No	• Language negatively loaded

Instrument	Scale	Domains	Recall period	Scalable	Comments
Celiac Disease DUX[33]	12 items, 5-faces scale	• Having CD • Communication • Diet	Unspecified – "how feeling these days" and "how feeling lately"	No	• Modified from DUX • Pediatric measure with parent and child versions • Available in many languages
Celiac Disease Questionnaire[34]	28 items, 7-point Likert scale	• Emotional problems • Social problems • Disease-related worries • Gastrointestinal symptoms	Past 2 wk	No	
Celiac Disease Assessment Questionnaire[27,28]	32 items, 5-point Likert scale	• Stigma • Dietary burden • Symptoms • Social isolation • Worries and concerns	Past 4 wk	Yes	• Scores scalable with dimension scores and an overall index (analogous to SF-36)

Abbreviations: GSRS, gastrointestinal symptoms rating scale; SF-36, short form-36.

a Developed in accordance with specifications outlined in US Food and Drug Administration 2009 Guidance for Industry "Patient-Reported Outcome Measures: Use in Medical Product Development to Support Labeling Claims."

been shown to be fairly responsive to therapeutic intervention in placebo-controlled trials.[24] However, the GSRS was developed primarily for functional gastrointestinal disorders and peptic ulcer disease, is not optimized for CD, and does not measure any extraintestinal symptoms.[25] Recently, several CD-specific PROs that incorporate intestinal and extraintestinal symptoms have been developed, including the Celiac Symptom Index,[26] the Celiac Disease PRO,[24] the Celiac Disease Assessment Questionnaire (CDAQ),[27,28] and the Celiac Disease Symptom Diary (see **Table 1**).[29]

Although symptom-based PROs have been suggested as a primary outcome in therapeutic trials for CD, there are several concerns. Fundamentally, the PROs described previously have been shown to be responsive to treatment and can detect statistical differences in symptom severity with a therapeutic intervention; however, the minimum clinically important difference has not been well-defined. As the smallest change in an outcome that a patient would identify as important, minimum clinically important difference offers a threshold above which an outcome is perceived as relevant by the patient. There is a need to establish consensus on change in CD-specific PRO scores that is perceived as minimum clinically important difference by patients. Another concern with symptom-based PROs in CD is the lack of correlation between symptoms and objective measures of CD activity. Thus, objective measures of disease activity, such as histology, should be included as coprimary or secondary outcomes in clinical trials for CD as described previously. In addition, most PROs were developed in adults and their applicability in children is not clear and no pediatric observer-reported outcomes have been validated.

PATIENT-REPORTED OUTCOMES FOR MEASUREMENT OF HEALTH-RELATED QUALITY OF LIFE

Although symptom-focused PROs are likely to be acceptable as a primary outcome in CD by regulatory agencies, HRQoL might arguably be a more important measure for patients. HRQoL in CD is determined not only by ongoing gastrointestinal and extraintestinal symptoms but also by high treatment burden because of psychological burden, social isolation, and financial challenges associated with a GFD. Any intervention, ether an adjunct or an alternative to a GFD, should aim to improve the psychological burden associated with accidental gluten exposure and social isolation related to a GFD without significantly increasing the economic burden of celiac patients, which is already high. An ideal HRQoL measure for CD should assess these aspects of quality of life. Given there are several aspects of HRQoL that are unique to CD, using a CD-specific HRQoL measure might provide insight into overall value of a therapeutic intervention in patients with CD. Several CD-specific HRQoL instruments have been validated for adult and pediatric patients with CD (see **Table 1**). The Celiac Disease Quality of Life Survey is the most extensively studied and assesses quality of life along four domains: (1) dysphoria, (2) inadequate treatment, (3) limitations, and (4) health concerns.[32] However, for each HRQoL measure, attention should be paid to individual domains in addition to overall score. For example, although a new therapy might improve the inadequate treatment domain through availability of more treatment options, it is still important to ensure that there is improvement (or at least no worsening) in other domains of Celiac Disease Quality of Life Survey with newer therapies.

Recently, a new instrument the CDAQ was developed.[27,28] It seems to be a hybrid of symptom-related PRO and HRQoL that assesses a variety of domains: symptoms, dietary burden, social isolation, stigma, and worry and concerns. Thus, CDAQ might be a simple to use and comprehensive measure of disease and treatment burden in patients with CD. However, there is a need to assess CDAQ responsiveness to change and develop more such instruments.

Although HRQoL is likely the most important outcome measure for patients, measurement of HRQoL in a randomized controlled setting might not be a true reflection of that in a clinical setting. This is because some of the factors inherent to a randomized controlled trial, such as more frequent interaction with patients, changes in dietary behavior of patients while in trial, and anxiety about side effects from a new therapy, bias patient population and confound HRQoL. Thus, although it is important to measure HRQoL in therapeutic trials, measuring HRQoL in more real-world settings is generally more relevant.

MEASURES OF SICKNESS BURDEN

In contrast to quality of life measures, burden of disease instruments are less well developed and less frequently used, but should be considered in CD. Two general categorizations of burden of disease are reported in the literature: the disability-adjusted life year (DALY), which was initially developed for the World Health Organization Global Burden of Disease survey,[35] and the quality-adjusted life year (QALY), which was developed by researchers at the University of York.[36]

The DALY measurement unit is used to quantify the burden of disease in specific populations, and is based on relevant health care costs.[37] The DALY includes years of "healthy" life lost because of death and years of "healthy" life lost because of poor health. DALY is considered an estimate of the difference between optimal health and the health of a specific population, such as individuals with CD. Whereas DALY measures the health loss, QALY measures the health gained. The QALY is able to combine the survival of an individual with their HRQoL into a single index, thereby providing a common currency to enable comparisons across different disease areas.[38] The main use of QALYs is within the framework of cost-effectiveness analysis, to assess the improvement in quality-adjusted life expectancy obtained through a specific health intervention relative to a situation in which either no intervention or a standard alternative intervention is provided.[39] In the current cost-sensitive environment, assessment of health care utilization is increasingly important. The need for understanding of health care utilization in CD is most commonly cited in discussions regarding population screening or payer considerations for emerging therapies. Money spent per QALY may be a key factor in determination of the acceptability of population screening initiatives, such as are considered necessary to significantly reduce the rate of undiagnosed CD.[40] Similarly, cost to the health care system to achieve meaningful improvements in either HRQoL or QALYs may be critical in payer acceptance of adjunctive therapies for CD.

DISCUSSION
Case Study: Dietary Interventions for Celiac Disease

Classically, diet-related interventions for patients with CD have focused on broadening the spectrum of grains considered suitable for a GFD, such as oats[41,42] or ancient wheat cultivars.[43] Educational (eg, CD school[44]), behavioral (eg, psychological support[45]), and technological (eg, testing for gluten in food, testing for gluten immunogenic peptides [GIPs] in urine or feces) interventions to improve GFD adherence have also been evaluated. As gluten-free processed foods have become more widely available, concerns regarding the nutritional quality of a GFD have increased.[46] Thus, we consider the case of a hypothetical trial comparing the Mediterranean diet to nutritional counseling to improve the nutritional profile of a GFD.

The primary challenge in assessing dietary interventions is the absence of an agreed-on measure of GFD adherence.[47] Classically, feeding studies have been conducted in inpatient settings where all food and beverages are provided and strictly controlled. Such an approach is less than ideal for dietary intervention studies in CD. Living in a controlled setting makes it difficult to measure the important dimension of how the intervention affects quality of life for an illness in which meal preparation and planning may be a considerable component of the treatment burden.[48–50] An alternative is to provide gluten-free meals through a home meal delivery service. Either preprepared meals or gluten-free ingredients to prepare meals could be provided. This approach has been used successfully in nutritional interventions for oncology patients, the elderly, and overweight teenagers.[51] Of course, provision of gluten-free food does not prevent gluten exposure entirely, either through inadvertent cross-contact during preparation and serving or through intentional ingestion and is not a sustainable practice outside of clinical trials.

For individuals sourcing their own meals, dietary assessment by a dietitian with expertise in GFDs is commonly accepted as the best available proxy for gluten exposure. Unfortunately, this method has not been standardized and is further limited by recall bias, patient knowledge of whether foods contain gluten,[52] and absence of symptoms to signal unintentional gluten exposure. More recently, tests for excretion of GIPs in stool[53] and urine[54] have been developed. These tests rely on the fact that human endoproteases are unable to cleave the prolyl peptide bonds of gluten.[55] Consequently, polypeptide fragments of 33 amino acids or longer may pass through the digestive system intact. Conveniently, these fragments are also immunogenic for many patients with CD.[55] The availability of assays to measure GIP excretion in urine and stool directly as a proxy for gluten ingestion has demonstrated gluten exposure that was not suspected following dietitian assessment[56] and an expert panel recently recommended that GIP testing be considered for use as a tool to select patients and/or document gluten exposure.[57]

Appropriate primary outcomes for dietary intervention studies must consider not only how the intervention affects dietary composition or adherence, but also the impact of this intervention on quality of life. Hypervigilance has been associated with decreased quality of life and emphasis on dietary adherence may also generate or exacerbate anxiety.[58] Thus, PROs may have a role either as a secondary or a coprimary end point.

Case Study: Pharmacologic Adjunct to a Gluten-Free Diet in Celiac Disease

Leffler and colleagues[24] reported a multicenter, randomized, double-blind, placebo-controlled study of larazotide acetate in adults with CD who had persistent symptoms despite at least 12 months of a GFD. A range of daily oral doses of Larazotide as adjunct to a GFD was evaluated over a 12-week period. Inclusion criteria were based on symptoms alone, thus it is unclear if the drug-effect varies with degree of histologic damage at the time of therapy. The primary end point was the difference in average weekly on-treatment CD-GSRS score for each dose versus placebo, over the 12-week active treatment period. This trial rightly chose a change in PRO score as the primary outcome. However, CD-GSRS was not developed in accordance with FDA regulatory guidelines and lacks assessment of extraintestinal symptoms related to CD. Although this trial included a change from baseline in celiac-specific PRO as a secondary outcome (this study also served as a validation exercise for celiac-specific PRO), future trials should use one of the validated, celiac-specific PROs specifically developed in accordance with FDA regulatory guidelines as a primary or coprimary outcome.

The trial also assessed serology at baseline and at several time-points during the study as safety measure. However, histologic assessment was not performed for this trial. Given the lack of correlation between serology and histology on a GFD, consideration should be given to include histology as coprimary or secondary end point. This trial also assessed GFD compliance using GFD compliance questionnaire and showed individuals on study drug and placebo reported similar rates of voluntary and accidental gluten consumption during the study period. Because diet question-naires are poor predictors of compliance, objective measures, such as GIP excretion, should be considered in future trials.

Case Study: Assessing Outcomes in Real-World Settings

Outcomes for real world studies may include the type of outcomes used in clinical tri-als, including gastrointestinal symptoms and histology, but are uniquely suited for assessment of critical variables including quality of life, burden of disease, and health care utilization.

Two classic real-world studies in CD by Johnston and colleagues[59] and Mustalahti and colleagues[60] assessed the effect of CD screening on quality of life in European populations. Although both studies assessed the effect of screening in similar popu-lations (mixed symptomatic and screen-detected adults detected by serologic tests) during a similar time period, the Johnston paper concluded "Quality of life in screen detected celiac patients did not differ significantly compared to controls." In contrast, the Mustalahti paper concluded "Gluten-free diet was associated with improved qual-ity of life for patients with symptom-detected CD and patients with screen-detected CD."

Although these studies are superficially similar, the primary outcomes differed. Johnston and colleagues[59] used the Short Form-36, whereas Mustalahti and col-leagues[60] used the Psychological General Well Being Index (PGWBI). It is probable that a major reason for the disparate conclusions is the choice of end point. Specif-ically, the Short Form-36 is heavily weighted to physical disability, whereas the PGWBI encompasses psychological, social, and emotional status. Given that the studies were both focused predominantly on the effect of CD diagnosis in screen detected, and thus pauci-symptomatic, individuals, the PGWBI was arguably the more appropriate and responsive choice. At the same time, the PGWBI lacks any questions that allow assessment of the relationships among disease, treatment, and symptoms on overall quality of life and thus would not currently be considered to be adequately represen-tative of the experience of living with CD. Although better measures currently exist, as described previously, these two real-world studies of CD diagnosis are helpful re-minders of the importance of choosing an appropriate primary outcome tailored for the specific population and study design in question.

SUMMARY

CD is a common condition that is underdiagnosed and for which the current treat-ments are inadequate and difficult. An unprecedented number of pharmacologic alter-natives to a GFD are currently under investigation, and studies of interventions to improve diagnosis and dietary treatment. A major challenge in any of these areas is designing appropriate trials with adequate outcome measures. Traditionally, investi-gators have relied on tissue transglutaminase antibodies and/or histology; however, these are poor proxies for either symptoms or HRQoL. The absence of a definitive cri-terion standard threatens to hinder progress in this area. Further work is necessary to establish outcome clinical measures for CD that are robust, relevant, responsive to treatment, noninvasive, and clinically meaningful. Such measures would include not only biomarkers of CD activity, but also PRO measures that can apply and be compared in the context of a gluten-free and a gluten-containing diet.

REFERENCES

1. Yan D, Holt PR. Willem Dicke. Brilliant clinical observer and translational investigator. Discoverer of the toxic cause of celiac disease. Clin Transl Sci 2009;2(6):446–8.
2. Rubio-Tapia A, Hill ID, Kelly CP, et al. ACG clinical guidelines: diagnosis and management of celiac disease. Am J Gastroenterol 2013;108(5):656–76 [quiz: 677].
3. Shah S, Akbari M, Vanga R, et al. Patient perception of treatment burden is high in celiac disease compared with other common conditions. Am J Gastroenterol 2014;109(9):1304–11.
4. Theethira TG, Dennis M, Leffler DA. Nutritional consequences of celiac disease and the gluten-free diet. Expert Rev Gastroenterol Hepatol 2014;8(2):123–9.
5. Leffler DA, Dennis M, Hyett B, et al. Etiologies and predictors of diagnosis in nonresponsive celiac disease. Clin Gastroenterol Hepatol 2007;5(4):445–50.
6. Singh P, Arora A, Strand TA, et al. Global prevalence of celiac disease: systematic review and meta-analysis. Clin Gastroenterol Hepatol 2018. https://doi.org/10.1016/j.cgh.2017.06.037.
7. Adelman DC, Murray J, Wu TT, et al. Measuring change in small intestinal histology in patients with celiac disease. Am J Gastroenterol 2018;113(3):339–47.
8. Corrao G, Corazza GR, Bagnardi V, et al. Mortality in patients with coeliac disease and their relatives: a cohort study. Lancet 2001;358(9279):356–61. Available at: http://www.ncbi.nlm.nih.gov/pubmed/11502314. Accessed March 19, 2013.
9. Rubio-Tapia A, Rahim MW, See JA, et al. Mucosal recovery and mortality in adults with celiac disease after treatment with a gluten-free diet. Am J Gastroenterol 2010;105(6):1412–20.
10. Lebwohl B, Granath F, Ekbom A, et al. Mucosal healing and mortality in coeliac disease. Aliment Pharmacol Ther 2013;37(3):332–9.
11. Silvester JA, Kurada S, Szwajcer A, et al. Tests for serum transglutaminase and endomysial antibodies do not detect most patients with celiac disease and persistent villus atrophy on gluten-free diets: a meta-analysis. Gastroenterology 2017;153(3):689–701.e1.
12. Leffler D, Schuppan D, Pallav K, et al. Kinetics of the histological, serological and symptomatic responses to gluten challenge in adults with coeliac disease. Gut 2013;62(7):996–1004.
13. Leffler D, Kupfer SS, Lebwohl B, et al. Development of celiac disease therapeutics: report of the third gastroenterology regulatory endpoints and advancement of therapeutics workshop. Gastroenterology 2016;151(3):407–11.
14. Adriaanse MPM, Leffler DA, Kelly CP, et al. Serum I-FABP detects gluten responsiveness in adult celiac disease patients on a short-term gluten challenge. Am J Gastroenterol 2016;111(7):1014–22.
15. Adriaanse MPM, Mubarak A, Riedl RG, et al. Progress towards non-invasive diagnosis and follow-up of celiac disease in children: a prospective multicentre study to the usefulness of plasma I-FABP. Sci Rep 2017;7(1):8671.
16. Morón B, Verma AK, Das P, et al. CYP3A4-catalyzed simvastatin metabolism as a non-invasive marker of small intestinal health in celiac disease. Am J Gastroenterol 2013;108(8):1344–51.

17. Tortora R, Capone P, De Stefano G, et al. Metabolic syndrome in patients with coeliac disease on a gluten-free diet. Aliment Pharmacol Ther 2015;41(4):352–9.
18. Ukkola A, Mäki M, Kurppa K, et al. Changes in body mass index on a gluten-free diet in coeliac disease: a nationwide study. Eur J Intern Med 2012;23(4):384–8.
19. Kabbani TA, Goldberg A, Kelly CP, et al. Body mass index and the risk of obesity in coeliac disease treated with the gluten-free diet. Aliment Pharmacol Ther 2012; 35(6):723–9.
20. Abu Daya H, Lebwohl B, Lewis SK, et al. Celiac disease patients presenting with anemia have more severe disease than those presenting with diarrhea. Clin Gastroenterol Hepatol 2013;11(11):1472–7.
21. U.S. Department of Health and Human Services Food and Drug Administration. Guidance for industry use in medical product development to support labeling claims guidance for industry. Clin Fed Regist 2009;1–39. https://doi.org/10.1111/j.1524-4733.2009.00609.x.
22. Daperno M, D'Haens G, Van Assche G, et al. Development and validation of a new, simplified endoscopic activity score for Crohn's disease: the SES-CD. Gastrointest Endosc 2004;60(4):505–12.
23. Taavela J, Kurppa K, Collin P, et al. Degree of damage to the small bowel and serum antibody titers correlate with clinical presentation of patients with celiac disease. Clin Gastroenterol Hepatol 2013;11(2):166–71.e1.
24. Leffler DA, Kelly CP, Green PHR, et al. Larazotide acetate for persistent symptoms of celiac disease despite a gluten-free diet: a randomized controlled trial. Gastroenterology 2015;148(7):1311–9.e6.
25. Svedlund J, Sjödin I, Dotevall G. GSRS: a clinical rating scale for gastrointestinal symptoms in patients with irritable bowel syndrome and peptic ulcer disease. Dig Dis Sci 1988;33(2):129–34. Available at: http://www.ncbi.nlm.nih.gov/pubmed/3123181.
26. Leffler DA, Dennis M, Edwards George J, et al. A validated disease-specific symptom index for adults with celiac disease. Clin Gastroenterol Hepatol 2009; 7(12):1328–34, 1334.e1-3.
27. Health Outcomes: The Coeliac Disease Assessment Questionnaire (CDAQ). Oxford University. Available at: https://innovation.ox.ac.uk/outcome-measures/coeliac-disease-assessment-questionnaire-cdaq/. Accessed June 8, 2018.
28. Crocker H, Jenkinson C, Churchman D, et al. The Coeliac Disease Assessment Questionnaire (CDAQ): development of a patient-reported outcome measure. Value Heal 2016;9:A595.
29. Murray JA, Kelly CP, Green PHR, et al. No difference between latiglutenase and placebo in reducing villus atrophy or improving symptoms in patients with symptomatic celiac disease. Gastroenterology 2017;152(4):787–98.e2.
30. Ware JE. SF-36 health survey update. Spine (Phila Pa 1976) 2000;25(24):3130–9. Available at: http://www.ncbi.nlm.nih.gov/pubmed/11124729.
31. Dupuy HJ. The psychological general well-being (PGWB) index. In: Wagner NK, Mattson ME, Fruberg CV, editors. Assessment of quality of life in clinical trials of cardiovascular therapies. New York: Le Jacq Publishing Inc; 1984. p. 170–83.
32. Dorn SD, Hernandez L, Minaya MT, et al. The development and validation of a new coeliac disease quality of life survey (CD-QOL). Aliment Pharmacol Ther 2010;31(6):666–75.
33. van Doorn RK, Winkler LMF, Zwinderman KH, et al. CDDUX: a disease-specific health-related quality-of-life questionnaire for children with celiac disease. J Pediatr Gastroenterol Nutr 2008;47(2):147–52.

34. Häuser W, Gold J, Stallmach A, et al. Development and validation of the Celiac Disease Questionnaire (CDQ), a disease-specific health-related quality of life measure for adult patients with celiac disease. J Clin Gastroenterol 2007;41(2): 157–66.

35. Murray CJL, Lopez AD. The global burden of disease: a comprehensive assessment of mortality and disability from deceases, injuries and risk factors in 1990 and projected to 2010, vol. 1. Cambridge (MA): Harvard University Press; 1996. p. 1–35.

36. Alexiou D. How the assessment of burden of illness might change NICE decisions: a retrospective analysis under value-based pricing. Athens J Heal 2014;115–28.

37. Murray CJ, Acharya AK. Understanding DALYs (disability-adjusted life years). J Health Econ 1997;16(6):703–30.

38. Whitehead SJ, Ali S. Health outcomes in economic evaluation: the QALY and utilities. Br Med Bull 2010;96(1):5–21.

39. Sassi F. Calculating QALYs, comparing QALY and DALY calculations. Health Policy Plan 2006;21(5):402–8.

40. Norstrom F, Lindholm L, Sandstrom O, et al. Delay to celiac disease diagnosis and its implications for health-related quality of life. BMC Gastroenterol 2011; 11(1):118.

41. Hoffenberg EJ, Haas J, Drescher A, et al. A trial of oats in children with newly diagnosed celiac disease. J Pediatr 2000;137(3):361–6.

42. Holm K, Mäki M, Vuolteenaho N, et al. Oats in the treatment of childhood coeliac disease: a 2-year controlled trial and a long-term clinical follow-up study. Aliment Pharmacol Ther 2006;23(10):1463–72.

43. Zanini B, Villanacci V, De Leo L, et al. Triticum monococcum in patients with celiac disease: a phase II open study on safety of prolonged daily administration. Eur J Nutr 2015;54(6):1027–9.

44. Jacobsson LR, Friedrichsen M, Göransson A, et al. Does a coeliac school increase psychological well-being in women suffering from coeliac disease, living on a gluten-free diet? J Clin Nurs 2011. https://doi.org/10.1111/j.1365-2702.2011. 03953.x.

45. Addolorato G, De Lorenzi G, Abenavoli L, et al. Psychological support counselling improves gluten-free diet compliance in coeliac patients with affective disorders. Aliment Pharmacol Ther 2004;20(7):777–82.

46. Pellegrini N, Agostoni C. Nutritional aspects of gluten-free products. J Sci Food Agric 2015;95(12):2380–5.

47. Hall NJ, Rubin G, Charnock A. Systematic review: adherence to a gluten-free diet in adult patients with coeliac disease. Aliment Pharmacol Ther 2009;30(4): 315–30.

48. Hallert C, Grännö C, Hultén S, et al. Living with coeliac disease: controlled study of the burden of illness. Scand J Gastroenterol 2002;37(1):39–42. Available at: http://www.ncbi.nlm.nih.gov/pubmed/19154566.

49. Sverker A, Hensing G, Hallert C. 'Controlled by food': lived experiences of coeliac disease. J Hum Nutr Diet 2005;18(3):171–80.

50. Zarkadas M, Dubois S, Macisaac K, et al. Living with coeliac disease and a gluten-free diet: a Canadian perspective. J Hum Nutr Diet 2013;26(1):10–23.

51. de Ferranti SD, Milliren CE, Denhoff ER, et al. Providing food to treat adolescents at risk for cardiovascular disease. Obesity (Silver Spring) 2015;23(10):2109–17.

52. Silvester JA, Weiten D, Graff LA, et al. Is it gluten-free? Relationship between self-reported gluten-free diet adherence and knowledge of gluten content of foods. Nutrition 2015;32(7–8):777–83.
53. Comino I, Real A, Vivas S, et al. Monitoring of gluten-free diet compliance in celiac patients by assessment of gliadin 33-mer equivalent epitopes in feces. Am J Clin Nutr 2012;95(3):670–7.
54. Moreno ML, Cebolla Á, Muñoz-Suano A, et al. Detection of gluten immunogenic peptides in the urine of patients with coeliac disease reveals transgressions in the gluten-free diet and incomplete mucosal healing. Gut 2017;66(2):250–7.
55. Shan L, Molberg Ø, Parrot I, et al. Structural basis for gluten intolerance in celiac sprue. Science 2002;297(5590):2275–9.
56. Comino I, Fernández-Bañares F, Esteve M, et al. Fecal gluten peptides reveal limitations of serological tests and food questionnaires for monitoring gluten-free diet in celiac disease patients. Am J Gastroenterol 2016;111(10):1456–65.
57. Ludvigsson JF, Ciacci C, Green PH, et al. Outcome measures in coeliac disease trials: the Tampere recommendations. Gut 2018. https://doi.org/10.1136/gutjnl-2017-314853. gutjnl-2017-314853.
58. Wolf RL, Lebwohl B, Lee AR, et al. Hypervigilance to a gluten-free diet and decreased quality of life in teenagers and adults with celiac disease. Dig Dis Sci 2018;63(6):1438–48.
59. Johnston SD, Rodgers C, Watson RGP. Quality of life in screen-detected and typical coeliac disease and the effect of excluding dietary gluten. Eur J Gastroenterol Hepatol 2004;16(12):1281–6. Available at: http://www.ncbi.nlm.nih.gov/pubmed/15618833.
60. Mustalahti K, Lohiniemi S, Collin P, et al. Gluten-free diet and quality of life in patients with screen-detected celiac disease. Eff Clin Pract 2002;5(3):105–13. Available at: http://www.ncbi.nlm.nih.gov/pubmed/12088289. Accessed February 4, 2012.

Celiac Disease in Asia

Govind K. Makharia, MD, DM, DNB[a],*, Carlo Catassi, MD[b,c]

KEYWORDS

- Epidemiology • Small intestine • India • China • Gluten

KEY POINTS

- Once thought to be uncommon, celiac disease is now emerging in many Asian countries; Asia is now at the center stage of celiac disease.
- The prevalence of celiac disease in Asian countries such as India, Turkey, Israel, Saudi Arabia, and Iran is as high as in rest of the world.
- There is a need to increase awareness about celiac disease among primary care physicians and specialists.
- The widespread availability of serologic tests, reliable gluten-free food, legislation for gluten labeling, training of dieticians, and creation of patient support groups are some of the unmet needs in Asia.

INTRODUCTION

Until recently, celiac disease (CD) was considered extremely uncommon in most Asian countries. Although patients with CD among immigrants of Asian descent had been described in Europe and North America many years ago[1,2] and occasional case reports from Asian countries were available in the scientific literature,[3,4] Asian patients presenting with celiac-like symptoms (chronic diarrhea, malnutrition, and abdominal distention, etc) were usually diagnosed as having tropical sprue or kwashiorkor in their native countries.[5–7] After sensitive and specific serologic CD biomarkers such as IgA class anti-tissue transglutaminase (tTG) antibodies became available, recent screening studies performed in different Asian countries, for example, in Turkey,[8] Iran,[9] and India,[10] have shown that CD is a common and often underdiagnosed disorder in Asia.

It is becoming clear that CD is a disorder as frequent in Asia (or at least in a large part of this continent) as in Europe and America. With a population of more than 4.4 billion,

Disclosure Statement: G.K. Makharia declare no conflict of interest. C. Catassi: Received Scientific Consultancy for Dr Schär.
[a] Department of Gastroenterology and Human Nutrition, All India Institute of Medical Sciences, Ansari Nagar, New Delhi 110029, India; [b] Department of Pediatrics, Center for Celiac Research, Università Politecnica delle Marche, Piazzale Martelli Raffaele, 8, Ancona, Ancona 60121, Italy; [c] Division of Pediatric Gastroenterology, Massachussets General Hospital, Boston, MA 33131, USA
* Corresponding author.
E-mail addresses: govindmakharia@gmail.com; govindmakharia@aiims.edu

gastro.theclinics.com

Asia Is probably the major reservoir of undiagnosed CD in the world. Spanning from Turkey to Japan and from Russia to Indonesia, the genetic, social, cultural, and nutritional heterogeneity of the Asian population is huge. Likewise, the epidemiology, disease awareness, and availability of diagnostic and treatment facilities for CD is extremely variable in the Asian continent. For all these reasons, there is currently a strong interest in the investigation of CD in Asia, from both of research and public health prospective.[11]

In this article, we review specific aspects related to the epidemiology, clinical presentation, and treatment of CD in Asian continent.

CELIAC DISEASE DETERMINANTS IN ASIA

In general, the frequency of CD largely depends on the distribution of the 2 major causal factors at the population level, that is, the consumption of gluten-containing cereals, particularly wheat, and the frequency of HLA-related predisposing genotypes, that is, HLA-DQ2 and -DQ8.

Wheat Consumption

Wheat consumption shows the largest world variability in the Asian continent. The domestication of modern wheat varieties, for example, *Triticum aestivum*, first took place 12,000 years ago in a Western Asia area (the so-called Fertile Crescent) including parts of Iraq, Syria, Lebanon, Jordan, and Israel. Not surprisingly then, wheat is nowadays a staple food in many Middle East and Asian countries.[12] At the same time, rice, the major gluten-free cereal, was also domesticated in Asia, specifically in the region of the Yangtze River valley in China, and then spread to Southeast and South Asia. Nowadays rice is a staple cereal in many Eastern Asian countries, for example, Japan, Indonesia, the Philippines, and Vietnam. In 2 of the largest Asian countries, that is, India and China, the role of wheat and rice in human nutrition shows a patchy distribution. A recent study in China showed that the consumption of wheat in the northern area is higher than in the southern area, where rice is the dietary staple; most of the rural households living in northern China consume more wheat than rice, except for the northeastern provinces, whereas rice is the staple diet for southern urban households.[10,13] In India, wheat is the staple cereal in the so-called celiac belt in Northwest India, including states such as Punjab, Haryana, Delhi, Rajasthan, Uttar Pradesh, Bihar, and Madhya Pradesh, whereas rice is the predominant cereal in Southern and Eastern India.[14]

The variability of cereal consumption doubtless influences the prevalence of CD in different areas of the Asian continent. However, a progressive Westernization of the diet is diffusely taking place in Asian countries, owing to increasing consumption of gluten-rich food such as pizza, pasta, and hamburgers. For instance, in China the per capita annual purchases of breads and steamed breads in urban households were 1.14 kg and 6.82 kg, respectively in 2001, and increased by 37.3% and 69.6%, respectively, between 1995 and 2001.[13] Given the direct relationship between gluten consumption at the population level and the risk of CD development, the prevalence of CD is expected to increase in the near future in many Asian countries, particularly in the Southeastern part of the continent.

Quantitative data on the individual consumption of gluten-containing cereals in Asian countries are not available; however, wheat/gluten intake can be estimated on the basis of the food supply data collected by the Food and Agriculture Organization.[15] Food supply surveys are conducted on a countrywide basis each year by almost every country in the world. These surveys provide data on food availability or disappearance rather than actual food consumption. Typically, the data are collected for the entire country and a per capita estimate is derived by dividing by the number of individuals in the country. These surveys provide a rough estimate of the amounts of foods consumed by the country's population. **Table 1** reports the wheat and wheat derivatives supply for selected Asian countries. Again, a clearcut decreasing gradient in wheat supply from Northwest to Southeast Asia is noticeable.

HLA Predisposing Haplotypes

As discussed elsewhere in detail in this book, some HLA haplotypes (DQ2 and/or DQ8) represent a necessary factor for CD development. Furthermore, different combinations of these HLA predisposing alleles influence the risk of disease; for example, subjects bearing a double copy of the DQ2 heterodimer have an odds ratio of 5.4 to develop CD, compared with the reference risk associated to any other HLA-DQ2 and/or -DQ8 haplotype.[16] Pioneer studies conducted in different Asian countries, particularly Turkey,[17] Iran,[18] and India[19] showed the same strong association between CD and HLA-DQ2 and/or -DQ8 genetic factor predisposing to CD. In Northern India, CD shows a strong association with the conserved HLA haplotype A26-B8-DR3-DQ2 (AH8.2) and the Ax-B21-DR3-DQ2 haplotypes.[19] These haplotypes differ from the European conserved HLA-AH8.1 haplotype (A1-B8-DR3-DQ2) at many loci (AH8.2 for instance carries the DRB3*02 allele), but not at the DQA1 and DQB1 loci, where both carry DQA1*05:01 and DQB1*02:01. This observation argues for the universal involvement of the DQA1*05:01/DQB1*02:01 heterodimer (DQ2) in the etiology of CD.[20]

In Asia, as well as any other geographic area, the prevalence of CD is directly related to the frequency of HLA-DQ2 and -DQ8 predisposing genotypes. Unfortunately, the frequency of all the different HLA-DQ2 and -DQ8 combinations predisposing to CD is largely unknown in most Asian countries. It is, however, possible to map the distribution in Asia of the DQB1*02:01 (DQ2), that is, the major CD predisposing gene, using data collected by the Allele Frequency Net Database (**Table 2**).[21] Interestingly, the DQ2 gene is widely diffused in Asian countries, but it is less common in some Eastern and Southeastern Asian countries and its frequency shows a direct correlation with the quantity of gluten-containing cereals consumed at the population level. This finding is particularly evident in India and China, 2 large countries showing variable within-country pattern of cereal consumption. In India, the HLA-DQ2 allele frequency is higher in the prevalently wheat-consuming Northern part (31.9%) than in the prevalently rice-consuming Southern part of India (12.8% for Piramalai Kallars and 9% for Yadavas).[19,22] Likewise, the frequency of the DQB1*0201 allele is higher in the northern Chinese than in the southern Chinese populations, and the consumption of wheat in the northern area is higher than in the southern area, where rice is a dietary staple.[13]

Colocalization of gluten consumption and HLA-DQ2 is a worldwide finding that is particularly evident in Asia. This observation has been labeled the evolutionary celiac paradox, because a lower HLA-DQ2 prevalence should be expected in wheat consuming populations owing to the negative selective pressure caused by a disease (CD) that was potentially lethal in the past. The parallel geographic distribution of gluten intake and HLA-DQ2 and DQ8 genotypes must be explained by different mechanisms, that is, a positive selection of HLA CD-predisposing genotypes in the past pushed by protection against diseases widely diffused after the agricultural revolution, for example, tuberculosis, leprosy, and dental caries.[23]

Table 1
Wheat supply (g/capita/d) for people living in Asian countries

Western Asia		Central Asia		Eastern Asia		South and Southeast Asia	
Country	Wheat Supply (g/capita/d)	Country	Wheat Supply (g/capita/d)	Country	Wheat Supply (g/capita/d)	Country	Wheat Supply (g/capita/d)
Turkey	467	Kazakhstan	253	China	173	Afghanistan	439
Georgia	359	Kyrgyzstan	354	Japan	123	Bangladesh	48
Azerbaijan	609	Tajikistan	358	Mongolia	341	India	166
Jordan	307	Turkmenistan	517	North Korea	59	Pakistan	311
Israel	304	Uzbekistan	465	South Korea	139	Viet Nam	29
Iran	420			Taiwan	139	Thailand	30
Saudi Arabia	245			Hong Kong	146	Indonesia	70
Yemen	302			Macau	155	Philippines	63

Data from Dalgic B, Sari S, Basturk B, et al, Turkish Celiac Study Group. Prevalence of celiac disease in healthy Turkish school children. Am J Gastroenterol 2011;106:1512–7.

Table 2
Prevalence the major HLA-related celiac disease–predisposing allele (DQB1*02) in Asian populations

Western Asia		Eastern Asia		South and Southeast Asia	
Country	DQB1*02 % Prevalence	Country	DQB1*02 % Prevalence	Country	DQB1*02 % Prevalence
Turkey	16–23	Russia	0–26	Thailand	6–13
Lebanon	10–20	Pakistan	21–40	Vietnam	5–11
Israel	18–39	India	0–26	Myanmar	3–15
Jordan	16–20	China	0–27	Indonesia	2–15
Iraq	21	Mongolia	6–28	Philippines	4
Iran	12–26	South Korea	0–10		
Saudi Arabia	35–36	Japan	0–1		

Data from Yachha SK. Celiac disease: India on the global map. J Gastroenterol Hepatol 2006;21:1511–3.

THE PREVALENCE OF CELIAC DISEASE IN ASIA

In recent years, several studies investigated the prevalence of CD in different Asian countries, including a systematic review and metaanalysis performed by one of us (G.M.).[24] This metaanalysis showed that the pooled seroprevalence of CD in Asia was 1.6% in 47,873 individuals based on positive anti-tTG antibody (Ab) and/or anti-endomysial antibodies (EMA). The pooled prevalence of biopsy-proven CD in Asia was 0.5% in 43,955 individuals. As expected, the prevalence of CD among women was higher than in men (0.5% vs 0.4%). The pooled prevalence of CD was 0.3% in Iran, 0.5% in Turkey, 0.6% in India, and 0.7% in Israel. The pooled prevalence of CD was significantly higher in Israel and India as compared with Iran.[24] Herein, we briefly summarize the major findings of the largest CD screening studies performed in Asian countries.

In Turkey, a large multicenter CD screening was performed on 20,190 school children between 2006 and 2008, by testing for IgA-tTG and total serum IgA, and EMA and intestinal biopsy in anti-tTG Ab-positive cases. The biopsy-proven prevalence of newly detected CD was 0.47% (1:212 children) in healthy Turkish school children, however, the estimated prevalence of CD, including biopsy-proven CD plus already diagnosed CD plus subjects with high anti-tTG Ab and EMA positivity without biopsy, was 1:58 (1.74%).[8] As for Iran, a metaanalysis of CD screening studies has recently been performed on 7 publications with 9720 subjects. Overall, the pooled prevalence of CD among the Iranian population was 0.72%. There was no significant heterogeneity among the studies. The pooled prevalence of CD on the basis of IgA anti-tTG Ab and anti-tTG Ab in combination of and presence of villus abnormalities on duodenal biopsy was 0.83% and 0.79%, respectively.[25] Large studies on the prevalence of CD in Russia have not been carried out yet, and the only detailed study presented in the international scientific literature focused on CD prevalence in Karelia, an area belonging to Northern Europe. In this study, the frequency of biopsy-proven CD was reported as 1:496.[26] In addition, a number of local publications can be found, which are only available in the Russian language. These reports contain scattered data from different regions of Russia, with the CD prevalence varying from 0.20% to 0.57% in the general population.[27]

A large CD screening study was recently performed in different parts of India. A total of 23,331 healthy adults were sampled from 3 regions of India—the northern part (n = 6207), the northeastern part (n = 8149), and the southern part (n = 8973) and screened for CD using IgA anti-tTG Ab. Positive tests were reconfirmed using a second enzyme-linked immunosorbent assay. CD was diagnosed if the second test was positive and these participants were further investigated. A subsample of participants was tested for HLA-DQ2/-DQ8 and underwent detailed dietary evaluation. The age-adjusted prevalence of celiac autoantibodies was 1.23% in northern India, 0.87% in northeastern India, and 0.10% in southern India. The prevalence of CD and potential CD, was 8.53 per 1000 in northern, 4.66 per 1000 in northeastern, and 0.11 per 1000 in the southern part respectively. The population prevalence of genes determining HLA-DQ2 and/or -DQ8 expression was 38.1% in northern, 31.4% in northeastern, and 36.4% in southern India. The mean daily wheat intake was highest in northern (455 g) compared with the northeastern (37 g) or southern parts (25 g), whereas daily rice intake showed an inverse pattern.[28] The high prevalence of the HLA-predisposing genotype (36.4%) in Southern India is at variance with previously reported data from this area and required confirmation from further studies.[19]

The epidemiology of CD in China was largely unknown until recent years. In a cross-sectional study, 19,778 undiagnosed Chinese adolescents and young adults (age 16–25 years) from 27 geographic regions in China were recruited at 2 universities in Jiangxi, China, from September 2010 through October 2013. All subjects were tested for IgG against deamidated gliadin peptides and IgA anti-tTG Ab. In general, the prevalence of CD autoimmunity was low in this Chinese population sample, although the prevalence seemed to vary among different areas in China. It was higher in northern provinces, such as Shandong, Shaanxi, and Henan, in which wheat was the dietary staple. The prevalence of CD autoimmunity in Shandong province was 0.76% (95% confidence interval, 0.21%–1.95%), similar to the world prevalence of CD. The prevalence of CD autoimmunity in populations form northern regions, where wheat is the staple diet, was 12 times higher than in populations from other regions, where rice is the staple diet.[29]

Reports from Malaysia, Japan, and Singapore suggest the existence of CD in Southeastern Asia; however, the prevalence of CD in this area is either very low or unknown. In, Japan an anti-tTG Ab based CD screening was recently performed on a sample from the general population (n = 2008). Although an unexpectedly high proportion of subjects showed anti-tTG Ab positivity (8%), none of them was EMA positive and only 1 showed celiac-type alterations on the small intestinal biopsy (CD prevalence of 0.05%).[30] It is worth noting that a very similar result was found in a recent anti-tTG Ab-based CD general screening performed on 1961 Vietnamese children: a high prevalence of tTG positivity (1%), with EMA negativity in all tTG positives and no case of CD.[31] It is not clear whether the high incidence of anti-tTG positive/EMA negative cases in these studies reflects a true different serologic phenotype, in comparison with Western populations, or merely represents a technical artifact. There are no formal reports on CD from Indonesia, Korea, Taiwan, or many other nations in this region.[32]

Table 3 summarizes the available information on CD prevalence in Asian countries/areas. CD is more common in countries/areas where gluten consumption is deeply rooted and HLA-predisposing genotypes are more diffused. This finding is perfectly logical, but still represents an evolutionary paradox waiting for an explanation.

THE CELIAC ICEBERG IN ASIA: LARGELY SUBMERGED

The ratio between the percentage of CD cases that are diagnosed on clinical ground and the overall CD prevalence (as determined by mass serologic screening) describes

Table 3 Estimated CD prevalence in different Asian countries			
High (Western Type) CD Prevalence ($\approx$ 1%)	Low CD Prevalence (0.1%–0.5%)	Very Low CD Prevalence (<0.1%)	Unknown CD Prevalence (Likely Very Low)
Turkey	Russia	Japan	Korea
Israel	China	Vietnam	Indonesia
Iran	India (South)		Malaysia
Saudi Arabia			Philippines
India (Northwest)			

Abbreviation: CD, celiac disease.

the burden of cases remaining clinically undetected, that is, the submerged part of the celiac iceberg. This estimation is influenced by doctors' awareness of the clinical variability of CD, the knowledge of CD among the general audience, the availability of diagnostic tools and gluten-free products.

Generally speaking, few data are available on the size of the "invisible" celiac iceberg. In an adult Jewish population screened in Israel for CD, the prevalence of CD diagnosed before recruitment was 0.12% and increased to 1.1% based on positive serology; that is, almost 90% of cases were clinically undetected.[33] In the previously cited large Turkish CD screening study,[8] the percentage of undiagnosed CD was only 45.5%, an outlier result compared not only with other Asian countries, but also with data from countries showing a strong tendency to unselective CD case finding, for example, Sweden and Italy.[34]

The picture is much more pessimistic in many other Asian countries, as shown by data from India. Based on several community-based CD screening studies, 5 to 8 million people are expected to have CD in India. Of such a large pool of patients, only a few thousand patients with CD have been diagnosed and a large number of subjects are still undiagnosed.[10] In other words, only a tiny portion of the overall number of CD cases have been diagnosed in India, roughly estimable as 0.125% to 0.200%. This finding means that a critical mass of patients exposed to the risk of long-term CD complications is left untreated. To the best of our knowledge no such data are available for many other Asian countries, for example, China and Eastern Russia, but there are reasons to believe that CD is largely undiagnosed in most wheat-consuming Asian populations.

SPECIFIC ISSUES FOR RECOGNITION AND MANAGEMENT OF CELIAC DISEASE IN ASIA
Measures to Increase Recognition of Celiac Disease in Asia

Broad strategies to increase recognition of CD in this region are described herein.

Establish the prevalence of celiac disease across Asia
Although tedious and labor intensive, the availability of reliable blood-based screening test such as anti-tTG Ab detection by enzyme-linked immunosorbent assay provides an excellent opportunity for estimation of a population-based prevalence of CD in a particular country/region. The general belief that CD does not occur or is uncommon in many Asian countries is an impediment to the initiation of a full-blown, population-based study in many countries. An alternative approach in such countries could be conducting pilot studies to estimate the prevalence of CD in some of the high-risk patient groups, for instance, patients with type 1 diabetes, chronic diarrhea, anemia, or

short stature where the prevalence of CD is several folds higher than the general population. If the existence of CD is confirmed by these pilot studies, population-based studies can be conducted at a later occasion. Furthermore, a multicenter epidemiologic effort aimed to measure the relevant parameters (level of gluten intake, frequency and pattern of CD-predisposing genotypes) could help to clarify the complex interplay between genetic and environmental factors leading to CD development in Asia.

Increase in education of health care professionals about celiac disease

It is essential that an awareness of and knowledge about CD and its disease associations increase among medical practitioners. The obvious groups to target are pediatricians, family physicians, internists, gastroenterologists, and histopathologists. However, it should be emphasized that CD may report to other medical specialists such as endocrinologists where patients present with short stature or type 1 diabetes, to hematologists with anemia, to rheumatologists with metabolic bone diseases, and to gynecologists with delay in menarche, secondary amenorrhea, or infertility.

Currently, a due emphasis is not placed on CD in the undergraduate and postgraduate medical curriculum. In the majority of the undergraduate and postgraduate textbooks of medicine, CD is generally dealt with in the chapters on malabsorption and only limited information about CD is provided. A due emphasis should be put on CD during undergraduate and postgraduate medical education. Furthermore, a constant reminder should be provided to physicians, internists, gastroenterologists, hematologists, and endocrinologists through continuing medical education programs.

Generally, primary care physicians and family physicians are the first contact of patients with CD. Therefore, empowering primary care and family physicians should play key role in increasing the detection of CD. Gastroenterologists in Asian countries can play a key role in increasing the awareness in their own countries about CD. Very often, histopathologists are not conversant with the handling and reporting of mucosal biopsies from patients suspected to have CD. Although specialist gastrointestinal pathologists may be consulted or slides sent for review, it is necessary for all pathologists to be trained in handling such biopsies and at least providing a preliminary report to the attending physician. With the estimated prevalence of CD in Asia, it is very unlikely that there would be a commensurate increase in gastrointestinal pathologists. Hence, general histopathologists in these countries would screen biopsies and referrals would be limited to difficult cases. Furthermore, histopathologists would be required to train and supervise technical staff handling such specimens. This training could be done by ensuring appropriate training during residency, after graduation, and during fellowships, as well as through continuing medical educational programs. Similarly, awareness should be created and adequate training should be provided to technical staff in handling and properly orienting biopsies before cutting the sections of the biopsies.

Increase in allocation of resources

Government and nongovernmental funding agencies should prioritize and allocate funds for research (epidemiologic and basic research) on CD. Furthermore, funding to make serologic tests more readily accessible will promote their use.

Asia at a cross roads of both underdiagnosis and overdiagnosis of celiac disease

At the present time, many Asian countries are at a cross roads of both underdiagnosis and overdiagnosis of CD. Of a pool of millions of patients suspected to have CD, only a proportion are diagnosed as having CD, even if they are symptomatic and are seeking medical attention because of lack of wide awareness of CD in Asia. In contrast, many patients are diagnosed to have CD based on rather inadequate evidences or just on the basis of a positive serology report. Many of them are not even explained properly about gluten-free diet.[35]

Issues Regarding Presentation of Celiac Disease

Although CD was thought to be a disease of the small intestine, it is now known that immune reaction to gluten peptide is not limited only to small intestine; in fact, it affects many other organs, including the skin (dermatitis herpetiformis), liver, and brain. CD is truly a multisystem disease. Awareness of the protean manifestations and presentations of CD, particularly the so-called atypical ones, is a major issue facing Asia. It compounds the lack of awareness of the disease itself within the population. A high degree of clinical suspicion is important for diagnosis of CD because the manifestations of CD vary widely and are not limited to the intestine.[36–39] Education of the medical communities across wide variety of specialties as well as during medical training, as discussed elsewhere in this article, is required.

Diagnostic Issues

Making a diagnosis of CD requires clinical suspicion usually followed by performance of a screening serologic test followed by diagnostic histologic assessment of the duodenal mucosa. Both serology and histopathology have challenges for the Asian populations.

Serologic tests

Currently, most celiac-specific serologic assay kits in Asia are imported from Europe/North America. Their diagnostic cutoff values of Ab concentrations have been determined based on Caucasian populations. With the difference and diversity in gluten ingestion and genetic background, the cutoff values for a positive test in Asia may not be similar to those reported in Caucasians. Therefore, there is a real need for the estimation of population specific cutoff values of serologic tests especially for anti-tTG Ab, and anti-deamidated gliadin peptide Ab. The other diagnostic aspects of serologic tests such as specificity, sensitivity, positive predictive values, and negative predictive values should also be determined in Asian populations.

Histopathology

Because of the occurrence of tropical enteropathy, small intestinal villi may be shorter in people from many Asian countries. Furthermore, there is lack of normative data on the crypt:villus ratio and normal intraepithelial lymphocyte counts per 100 enterocytes, both of which are critical for making a diagnosis of CD. There is a need to define the cutoff values that identify intraepithelial lymphocytosis.

A firm diagnosis of CD should be made before initiating gluten-free diet in Asia because CD is a lifelong disease that requires lifelong therapy with a diet that is challenging. Furthermore, making a diagnosis of CD in patients already after a GFD has issues because the serologic and histologic criteria depend on the presence of pathogenic events related to gluten ingestion. In the current data, anti-tTG-2 Ab is the preferred screening test in those suspected to have CD.[40–42] For those who are IgA deficient, an IgG-based test is needed and anti-deamidated gliadin peptide seems to perform the best, at least in Caucasian populations. It is inappropriate to rely only on serology for diagnosis, especially with the uncertainties regarding interpretation of serologic tests in Asian populations. Hence, duodenal biopsies, including several biopsies of the first and second/third parts of the duodenum, are essential to secure the diagnosis.

Management Issues

Lifelong adherence to gluten-free diet is the cornerstone of successful disease management. There are many impediments to the institution of a successful gluten-free diet; some of them are universal and some of them are unique to many Asian countries. Patients with CD are challenged with barriers in the maintenance of a strict gluten-free diet because of factors such as inadequate information and education about the disease, widespread unavailability of reliable gluten-free food, and inadequate/no food labeling on the packaged food items.[38,43]

Training of dieticians

Successful management of CD requires a team approach, including patient, family, physicians, and dieticians. After a diagnosis is made, all patients should be referred to a dietician for nutritional assessment, diet education, meal planning, and assistance with the social and emotional adaptation to a gluten-free lifestyle. The management of CD is very different from that of other gastrointestinal diseases in that the core of the treatment is dietary and nonmedicinal.[44,45] Prescribing a gluten-free diet after diagnosis is easy, but its institution and maintenance of adherence pose the real challenges. Most physicians may not have enough expertise in counseling for gluten-free diet. In Western countries, dietitians play a pivotal role in the management of patients with CD. However, there is a lack of trained dietitians in most Asian nations; and even if they are there, most do not have sufficient expertise in the management of CD.

The dietary counselor should have sufficient knowledge about the GF food and food products. It is not only about prescribing gluten-free diet, but also is to provide an individual patient specific, well-balanced diet. Dieticians have academic and practical experience including in-depth knowledge regarding nutritional needs, nutrition composition, and socioeconomic, psychological, and educational factors that affect the food and nutrition behavior of people. They also have skills to translate scientific information into laymen's terms and assist individuals in gaining knowledge, and improving decision making. Although other health care professionals can disseminate nutrition advice, they do not have the training in nutrition sciences and food composition to be able to translate complex medical nutrition concepts and issues into attainable dietary changes.[46–49]

A delay in referral, or no referral at all, increases the likelihood of the patient obtaining inaccurate information from the Internet, health food stores, alternative health practitioners, and other sources, which may be outdated, inaccurate, and/or conflicting. Poorly informed patients might unnecessarily restrict certain foods, thus limiting the variety and nutritional quality of their diet.[48]

The need for gluten-free food infrastructure in the food supply chain Because of the perception that CD is uncommon and there exists a low absolute number of patients with CD, the need for industrial production of gluten-free diet has not been perceived in Asia. At present, there is neither an organized sector nor industry for gluten-free products in Asia, and gluten-free food products are not readily available. Although the number of patients with CD is small at present in Asia, there is a likelihood of an exponential increase in the number of patients with CD with increasing awareness about the disease, and hence the demand of gluten-free diet is likely to increase in the near future. Therefore, there is need for large-scale, industrial-level production of reliable and affordable gluten-free food, including choices of food products ranging from snacks, flour, sweets, ice creams, and ready-to-eat choices. The availability of gluten-free foods is one of the important determinants of dietary adherence.

Facility for gluten testing laboratories Before releasing for patient's use, all the gluten-free food products should be tested for their quality. In fact, there should be certified gluten checking laboratories where food items may be checked for their gluten contents. This step is important to ensuring the quality of food for its gluten content until the gluten-labeling legislation is enforced.

Legislation for gluten labeling Although the Food Safety and Standard Authority of India has laid down the standards for gluten-free food in India, many Asian countries should take steps in this regards. The Food Safety and Standard Authority of India has also made it mandatory for labeling of food items as to whether they contain gluten or they are gluten free.

SUMMARY

CD is emerging in many Asian nations. Although the absolute number of patients with CD at present is not very high, this number is expected to increase markedly over the next few years/decades owing to heightened awareness and increased diagnosis. It is now that the medical community across the Asia should define the extent of the problem and be preparing to handle the impending epidemic of CD in Asia.

REFERENCES

1. Walker-Smith JA. Coeliac disease in children of Asian immigrants. Lancet 1973; 1(7800):428.
2. Nelson R, McNeish AS, Anderson CM. Coeliac disease in children of Asian immigrants. Lancet 1973;1(7799):348–50.
3. Walia BN, Mehta S, Gupte SP. Coeliac disease. Indian Pediatr 1972;9:16–9.
4. Walia BN, Sidhu JK, Tandon BN, et al. Coeliac disease in North Indian children. Br Med J 1966;2:1233–4.
5. Baker SJ, Mathan VI. Tropical enteropathy and tropical sprue. Am J Clin Nutr 1972;25:1047–55.
6. Mehta SK. Clinical features and aetiopathogenesis of tropical sprue. J Assoc Physicians India 1971;19:417–24.
7. Misra RC, Chuttani HK. Prevalence of tropical sprue in a hospital population in North India. Ann Trop Med Parasitol 1969;63:117–22.
8. Dalgic B, Sari S, Basturk B, et al, Turkish Celiac Study Group. Prevalence of celiac disease in healthy Turkish school children. Am J Gastroenterol 2011;106: 1512–7.
9. Shahbazkhani B, Mohamadnejad M, Malekzadeh R, et al. Coeliac disease is the most common cause of chronic diarrhoea in Iran. Eur J Gastroenterol Hepatol 2004;16:665–8.
10. Makharia GK, Verma AK, Amarchand R, et al. Prevalence of celiac disease in the northern part of India: a community-based study. J Gastroenterol Hepatol 2011; 26:894–900.
11. Makharia GK, Mulder CJ, Goh KL, et al, World Gastroenterology Organization and Asia Pacific Association of Gastroenterology Working Party on Celiac Disease. Issues associated with the emergence of coeliac disease in the Asia–Pacific region: a working party report of the World Gastroenterology Organization and the Asian Pacific Association of Gastroenterology. J Gastroenterol Hepatol 2014;29:666–77.

12. Rostami K, Malekzadeh R, Shahbazkhani B, et al. Coeliac disease in Middle Eastern countries: a challenge for the evolutionary history of this complex disorder? Dig Liver Dis 2004;36:694–7.
13. Yuan J, Gao J, Li X, et al. The tip of the "celiac iceberg" in China: a systematic review and meta-analysis. PLoS One 2013;8:e81151.
14. Yachha SK. Celiac disease: India on the global map. J Gastroenterol Hepatol 2006;21:1511–3.
15. Food and Agriculture Organization of the United Nations. Food supply: crops primary equivalent. Available at: http://www.fao.org/faostat/en/#data/CC. Accessed May 1, 2018.
16. De Silvestri A, Capittini C, Poddighe D, et al. HLA-DQ genetics in children with celiac disease: a meta-analysis suggesting a two-step genetic screening procedure starting with HLA-DQ β chains. Pediatr Res 2018;83:564–72.
17. Erkan T, Kutlu T, Yilmaz E, et al. Human leukocyte antigens in Turkish pediatric celiac patients. Turk J Pediatr 1999;41:181–8.
18. Rostami-Nejad M, Romanos J, Rostami K, et al. Allele and haplotype frequencies for HLA-DQ in Iranian celiac disease patients. World J Gastroenterol 2014;20: 6302–8.
19. Kaur G, Sarkar N, Bhatnagar S, et al. Pediatric celiac disease in India is associated with multiple DR3-DQ2 haplotypes. Hum Immunol 2002;63:677–82.
20. Sollid LM. The roles of MHC class II genes and post-translational modification in celiac disease. Immunogenetics 2017;69:605–16.
21. Allele*Frequencies in Worldwide Populations. The allele frequency net database. Available at: www.allelefrequencies.net. Accessed May 1, 2018.
22. Shanmugalakshmi S, Balakrishnan K, Manoharan K, et al. HLA-DRB1, -DQB1 in two Dravidian-speaking castes of Tamil Nadu, South India. Tissue Antigens 2003; 61:451–64.
23. Lionetti E, Catassi C. Co-localization of gluten consumption and HLA-DQ2 and –DQ 8 genotypes, a clue to the history of celiac disease. Dig Liver Dis 2014; 46:1057–63.
24. Singh P, Arora S, Singh A, et al. Prevalence of celiac disease in Asia: a systematic review and meta-analysis. J Gastroenterol Hepatol 2016;31:1095–101.
25. Ahadi Z, Shafiee G, Razmandeh R, et al. Prevalence of celiac disease among the Iranian population: a systematic review and meta-analysis of observational studies. Turk J Gastroenterol 2016;27:122–8.
26. Kondrashova A, Mustalahti K, Kaukinen K, et al. Lower economic status and inferior hygienic environment may protect against celiac disease. Ann Med 2008;40: 223–31.
27. Savvateeva LV, Erdes SI, Antishin AS, et al. Overview of celiac disease in Russia: regional data and estimated prevalence. J Immunol Res 2017;2017:2314813.
28. Ramakrishna BS, Makharia GK, Chetri K, et al. Prevalence of adult celiac disease in India: regional variations and associations. Am J Gastroenterol 2016;111: 115–23.
29. Yuan J, Zhou C, Gao J, et al. Prevalence of celiac disease autoimmunity among adolescents and young adults in China. Clin Gastroenterol Hepatol 2017;15: 1572–9.
30. Fukunaga M, Ishimura N, Fukuyama C, et al. Celiac disease in non-clinical populations of Japan. J Gastroenterol 2018;53:208–14.
31. Zanella S, De Leo L, Nguyen-Ngoc-Quynh L, et al. Cross-sectional study of coeliac autoimmunity in a population of Vietnamese children. BMJ Open 2016; 6:e011173.

32. Makharia GK. Celiac disease screening in southern and East Asia. Dig Dis 2015; 33:167–74.
33. Israeli E, Hershcovici T, Grotto I, et al. Prevalence of celiac disease in an adult Jewish population in Israel. Isr Med Assoc J 2010;12:266–9.
34. Catassi C, Lionetti E. Case finding for celiac disease is okay, but is it enough? J Pediatr Gastroenterol Nutr 2013;57:415–7.
35. Vohra P. India should worry about underdiagnosis and overdiagnosis of coeliac disease. BMJ 2014;348:g2046.
36. Sainsbury A, Sanders DS, Ford AC. Prevalence of irritable bowel syndrome-type symptoms in patients with celiac disease: a meta-analysis. Clin Gastroenterol Hepatol 2013;11:359–65.
37. Aziz I, Sanders DS. The irritable bowel syndrome-celiac disease connection. Gastrointest Endosc Clin N Am 2012;22:623–37.
38. Haines ML, Anderson RP, Gibson PR. Systematic review: the evidence base for long-term management of coeliac disease. Aliment Pharmacol Ther 2008;28: 1042–66.
39. Kochhar R, Jain K, Thapa BR, et al. Clinical presentation of celiac disease among pediatric compared to adolescent and adult patients. Indian J Gastroenterol 2012;31:116–20.
40. Husby S, Koletzko S, Korponay-Szabó IR, et al, ESPGHAN Working Group on Coeliac Disease Diagnosis, ESPGHAN Gastroenterology Committee, European Society for Pediatric Gastroenterology, Hepatology, and Nutrition. European Society for Pediatric Gastroenterology, Hepatology, and Nutrition guidelines for the diagnosis of coeliac disease. J Pediatr Gastroenterol Nutr 2012;54:136–60.
41. Bai JC, Fried M, Corazza GR, et al, World Gastroenterology Organization. World Gastroenterology Organisation global guidelines on celiac disease. J Clin Gastroenterol 2013;47:121–6.
42. Rubio-Tapia A, Hill ID, Kelly CP, et al, American College of Gastroenterology. ACG clinical guidelines: diagnosis and management of celiac disease. Am J Gastroenterol 2013;108:656–76.
43. Hall NJ, Rubin G, Charnock A. Systematic review: adherence to a gluten-free diet in adult patients with coeliac disease. Aliment Pharmacol Ther 2009;30:315–30.
44. See J, Murray JA. Gluten-free diet: the medical and nutrition management of celiac disease. Nutr Clin Pract 2006;21:1–15.
45. García-Manzanares A, Lucendo AJ. Nutritional and dietary aspects of celiac disease. Nutr Clin Pract 2011;26:163–73.
46. Olsson C, Hörnell A, Ivarsson A, et al. The everyday life of adolescent coeliacs: issues of importance for compliance with the gluten-free diet. J Hum Nutr Diet 2008;21:359–67.
47. Nasr I, Leffler DA, Ciclitira PJ. Management of celiac disease. Gastrointest Endosc Clin N Am 2012;22:695–704.
48. Niewinski MM. Advances in celiac disease and gluten-free diet. J Am Diet Assoc 2008;108:661–72.
49. Case S. The gluten-free diet: how to provide effective education and resources. Gastroenterology 2005;128:S128–34.

The Microbiome in Celiac Disease

Suneeta Krishnareddy, MD, MS

KEYWORDS

- Microbiome • Celiac disease • Probiotics • Prebiotics

KEY POINTS

- The microbiome is vital for normal immune cell function and development.
- Alterations in the microbiome, or dysbiosis, is associated with celiac disease, as well as many other diseases.
- The microbiome is an important target for therapeutic potential in celiac disease.
- Prebiotics and probiotics are being studied as potential therapies in celiac disease, but further studies need to be done to elucidate their role.

INTRODUCTION

The human gastrointestinal tract is a complex and dynamic environment, sheltering a vast number and variety of commensal microorganisms.[1] This balanced microecosystem provides a natural defense against invasion of pathogens. Recently, much research has focused on the role of the human microbiome in health and disease, and the ability to harness the power of the human microbiome for treatment of these diseases.

Celiac disease (CD) is a complex multifactorial disorder involving both genetic and environmental factors. For many years, the only securely established genetic factors contributing to CD risk were various genetic variants located within the HLA region (those encoding the HLA-DQ2/DQ8 heterodimers).[2] With the introduction of genome-wide association studies and the immunochip study, an additional 39 non-HLA regions of susceptibility have been associated with CD development, some of which share with other autoimmune diseases.[3] Interestingly, most of the chromosome regions associated with CD predisposition contain genes with immune-related functions, and some CD susceptibility genes play a role in bacterial colonization and sensing. Studies also have shown an altered expression of nonspecific CD-risk genes involved in host-microbiota interactions in the intestinal mucosa of patients with CD,

Disclosure Statement: No financial disclosures.
Digestive and Liver Diseases, Columbia University, 180 Fort Washington, New York, NY 10032, USA
E-mail address: Sk3222@cumc.columbia.edu

Gastroenterol Clin N Am 48 (2019) 115–126
https://doi.org/10.1016/j.gtc.2018.09.008
0889-8553/19/© 2018 Elsevier Inc. All rights reserved.

such as those of toll-like receptors and their regulators.[4] Disturbances in the host-microbiota interaction and shifts in the immune balance in subjects with CD might propagate the inflammatory response by gluten, which is pathognomonic to CD.[5]

NORMAL COLONIZATION AND ITS IMPACT ON HUMAN DEVELOPMENT

Initial colonization of the infant gut by microbes sets the stage for the lifelong, relatively stable adult microbiome. Infants rely on colonization to complete development of the immune system and gastrointestinal tract. The first days and weeks of life represent a crucial window of opportunity for shaping the development of the gastrointestinal tract and immune system, as well as the future adult microbiome. "Normal colonization" likely affords protection of developing childhood and adult diseases. The evidence of the contribution of the microbiome to healthy immunity and defense against multiple diseases is growing, as the list includes many nonintestinal diseases, such as obesity, food allergies, and diabetes mellitus, in addition to intestinal-related autoimmune disorders, such as inflammatory bowel disease and CD.

In vaginal birth, the infant is inoculated as he or she passes through the birth canal. This inoculum is a mixture of gram-negative and gram-positive bacteria, aerobes, and anaerobes. This initial colonizing species has been shown to be important in establishing a "pioneer microbiome" that in turn educates the developing immune system and provides favorable conditions for colonization by subsequent microbes.[6]

Beneficial infant colonization is dependent on the maternal microbiota, which in turn is influenced by maternal genetics, environmental exposures, and diet before and during pregnancy as well as during breast-feeding. Once the infant has been inoculated, compounds already present in the infant gut as well as from breast milk act as prebiotics and encourage growth of commensals. Priming for microbial colonization begins in utero. The vernix caseosa, the waxy skin coating of a fetus, is shed into the amniotic fluid as the fetus approaches term. While still in utero, the fetus swallows amniotic fluid containing pieces of vernix. The vernix is made up of short-chain fatty acids (SCFAs) and lipids. Although these SCFAs and lipids are indigestible by human enzymes, they provide a rich medium for growth of bacteria. These prebiotics continue to be administered to the infant in the case of breast-feeding. Colostrum contains especially high concentrations of human milk oligosaccharides (HMOs), which are indigestible by human enzymes, but like the vernix SCFAs, promote growth of intestinal microbes.[7] The HMOs selectively promote growth of commensals, such as Bifidobacterium longus subspecies infantis, and suppress growth of pathogens, like Escherichia coli and Clostridium perfringens. Furthermore, growth of these bacteria on HMOs alters their activity, making Bifidobacterium infantis more bound to intestinal epithelial cells, which then affords a stronger barrier promoting an anti-inflammatory effect.[8] These prebiotics give commensals an advantage over pathogens in the developing infant gut, which helps prevent newborn enteric infections, as well as laying the foundation for a strong immune system.[9]

NORMAL COLONIZATION MAINTAINS HOMEOSTASIS OF THE IMMUNE SYSTEM

The microbiota play a role in shaping the architecture of the immune system (such as Peyer patches), the development of specific immune cell populations (such as regulatory T cells) and the balance between immune cell types. The 2 features of the gastrointestinal immune architecture most affected by microbiota are the mucous layer and gut-associated lymphoid tissue (GALT), which includes Peyer patches.[10]

The mucous layer maintains spatial segregation between the bacteria-rich gut lumen and the intestinal epithelium. This bacteria-free zone (approximately 50-μm thick) protects against otherwise continuous immune stimulation and inflammation. This segregation serves to augment the barrier function of the epithelial layer, which is only 1 single cell thick.[11] Intestinal microbes provide the stimuli for maintenance of the mucous layer. Germ-free animals have thinner mucous layer than conventional animals, with specific members of the microbiome contributing to production of mucous, such as *Akkermansia muciniphila* and *Lactobacillus* species.[12]

The innate immune system maintains the sterility of the mucous layer. Intestinal epithelial cells produce antibacterial RegIIIγ in an MyD88-dependent manner. RegIIIγ is an antibacterial C-type lectin that targets gram-positive bacteria. RegIIIγ knockout mice exhibited increased adaptive immune activation, increased fecal immunoglobulin (Ig)A and increased Th1 cells in the lamina propria. These increases were dependent on the intestinal microbiota. This physical segregation of the microbiota from the intestinal epithelium is an example by which the innate immune system maintains tolerance of the intestinal microbiota by limiting contact with the adaptive immune system.[13]

A healthy microbiome further protects the host by forming its own protection against colonization, a phenomenon known as colonization resistance. As mentioned previously, microbes stimulate the mucous layer and also stimulate the epithelium to secrete antimicrobial peptides into the mucous layer, providing a barrier against pathogens.[14] Commensals themselves can produce substances to prevent infections, such as acetate production by *Bifidobacterium*, which protects agaln enterohemorrhagic *E coli* O157:H7.[15]

In addition to the microbiome's effect on the physical barrier promoting immune tolerance, the microbiota also stimulates the formation of GALT. It has been shown that germ-free animals have dramatically reduced germinal centers in the GALT, and reduced secretory IgA.[16,17] IgA produced by the GALT acts in an immunomodulatory manner. Intestinal dendritic cells sample the intestinal lumen; when they come in contact with bacterial polysaccharide A (PSA), a component of the commensal *Bacteroides fragilis*, they then stimulate the adaptive immune response to secrete IgA, locally. This locally produced IgA then coats the bacterial antigen, resulting in decreased activation of the innate immune response.[18] In this way, GALT functions as a self-contained immune system, recognizing bacterial antigens and stimulating the immune response, but the response is contained to the mucosal compartment, thereby avoiding systemic inflammation. A study done in Swedish infants showed that increased diversity of *Bifidobacterium* species is associated with increased IgA,[19] which has been linked to protection against allergy and autoimmunity.[20]

These data support the role of the initial microbiome and "beneficial" bacteria in regulating the adaptive and innate responses.

MICROBIOTA BALANCE AND IMMUNE RESPONSES

The rapid colonization after birth shifts the perinatal immune system of that of hyperstimulation to that of tolerance. In this system, the neonatal gut allows colonization by microbes and a specific population of CD71+ erythroid cells dampens the innate immune response.[21] In addition to anti-inflammatory signals from the host, these signals also come from the colonized microbiota. SCFAs produced by host bacteria affect regulatory T-cell (T_{reg}) populations.[15] Butyrate (a commonly produced SCFA) increases the differentiation of progenitor cells to become T_{reg} cells, and SCFAs, in general, specifically expand the population of colonic T_{reg} cells.[22]

The microbiota also plays a key role in regulating the balance between populations of CD4+ helper T cells, Th1 and Th2 cells. During the perinatal period, the immune system is skewed toward a Th2 cytokine milieu; however, persistence of this Th2 environment has been associated with atopic diseases. This shift is caused by a bacterially derived carbohydrate. Gut dendritic cells protruding through the intestinal epithelium sample commensal B fragilis from the gut lumen; this sampled PSA is transported to the systemic immune system where it restores the balance between Th1 and Th2 cells.[23] It has been considered that the onset of CD is mediated by a skewed Th1 response. Although the exact cause of this skewed response is unknown, it can be suggested that the balance of these CD4+ cell subsets depends on a balanced microbiome.[24]

Similarly, Th17 cells, which are mostly proinflammatory cells that protect against infection at the mucosal surfaces, are also regulated by the microbiota, specifically, Th17 cells are induced by segmented filamentous bacteria (SFB).[25] In mice, SFB act via major histocompatibility complex class II (MHC-II) on intestinal dendritic cells to increase differentiation of CD4+ T cells into Th17 cells in the lamina propria.[26] These Th17 cells, which have been shown to have critical functions in host defense against bacterial pathogens and the inflammatory response to deamidated gliadin peptides, are important in the pathogenesis of CD.[27]

Through appropriate colonization and the resulting "education" of the gastrointestinal immune system, infants develop more optimal gut function. This early priming of the immune system is critical for later life. Dysbiosis is abnormal colonization, or the imbalance of microbes inhabiting a certain part of the body. The 4 known categories promoting intestinal dysbiosis are (1) abnormal microbial exposures, (2) disruptions in diet, (3) antibiotic usage and other medications, and (4) influence of host genetics.

Abnormal microbial exposures can occur at time of delivery, such as cesarean versus vaginal delivery. A study done in 2010 showed that infants born via vaginal delivery closely resembled their mother's vaginal microbiota, whereas those born via cesarean delivery reflected the microbes present in the infant's environment (including Staph).[6] Infants born via cesarean specifically lack presence of and diversity within the Bacteroidetes phylum. Although it is unclear if this is the cause of increased CD seen in children born via cesarean, this association has been made.[28,29] Many studies have focused on the association between microbial colonization and disease later in life, such as obesity, asthma, and allergy, and have found that the timing of colonization is also important. These data demonstrate the importance of a "window of opportunity" for microbial education of the developing immune system, which results in persistent alteration in systemic gene expression and, potentially, persistent changes in microbial populations.[30,31]

A possible second window of development for the intestine and immune system, especially regarding oral tolerance, is the exposure to dietary antigens. Data regarding the timing of antigen introduction to reduce likelihood of an autoimmune or allergic reaction are not uniform. In the case of CD, it is often stated that gluten should not be introduced before 4 months of age and not after 6 months of age. However, a small study done showed that the delayed introduction of gluten from 6 months to 12 months resulted in a decrease in the incidence of CD, as well as the development of anti-gliadin IgG antibodies.[29]

The effects of antibiotics and infections on the intestinal microbiome provide further evidence for the importance of a diverse microbiome in maintaining homeostasis, particularly in the perinatal period. A recent study in mice demonstrated that early antibiotic usage had a lasting effect on immunity and metabolism, even though changes in the microbiome were transient. Mice treated with antibiotics early in life were seen to have elevated fat mass and decreased expression of immune-related genes despite normalization of the microbiome.[31] In children and adults with HLA predisposition for CD, a gastrointestinal infection increased the risk of CD autoimmunity by 33%.[32] Another study done looking at the role of viral infections and initiation of Th1 cells, identified reovirus as a possible trigger for both the altered immune response seen in CD, as well as a factor in gliadin antigen tolerance.[33] These data highlight the importance of not only initial colonization but maintenance of "healthy" microbes in preventing disease development.

Studies of the role the microbiome in CD are evolving, and as with most studies of the microbiome, most studies have shown descriptive data, but lack cause and effect. Indeed, although CD is prevalent in both adults and children, most of the microbiome data in CD comes from studies done in children.[34–37] Studies characterizing the microbiota of adult patients with CD began only in 2012, and a single study of both children and adults reported a slight difference in the percentages of the main phyla between subjects and also a more diverse profile in duodenal biopsy specimens from adults.[38] The Firmicutes are the most abundant bacteria in adults with CD, whereas Proteobacteria are present mainly in children with CD. Other phyla shared between adults with CD and children with CD belong to the Bacteroidetes and Actinobacteria. Regarding bacterial genera, adults with CD harbor larger numbers of Mycobacterium spp and Methylobacterium spp, whereas Neisseria spp and Haemophilus spp are more abundant in children with CD. Although these studies have given us information about the general makeup of the microbiome of patients with CD, they do little to answer the questions if these changes precede disease onset, if they are a consequence of inflammation, or if the changes seen in the microbiome are associated with changes in immune cell phenotype. Future studies need to focus on causality, and possibly a specific bacterial group that could be pathogenic or protective in this group of patients, and that could be targeted for treatment.

Although it is unclear whether the altered microbiome is a cause of or consequence of disease, it is hypothesized that gram-negative bacteria in genetically susceptible individuals may contribute to the loss of gluten tolerance. If modified bacteria are a result of disease, the disrupted mucosa inundated with immature enterocytes could lead to conditions favoring gram-negative instead of gram-positive bacterial colonization. Although this theory has not been proven, early studies have shown a propensity toward higher gram-negative colonization in duodenal samples of pediatric patients with CD compared with healthy controls, in which case the dysbiosis seen seems to be of importance.[38] CD offers a unique disease in which to study the microbiome, as many other factors can be controlled for, including genetic makeup, environment, and triggers, as these are all known, and the effect of the microbiome on disease pathogenesis can be further explored. Also, because the genetic makeup can be determined before a subject acquires CD, it is possible to do longitudinal studies in these patients and observe the change in microbiome to see if the alterations noted are a cause of or consequence of disease.[39,40]

MICROBIOME AS A THERAPEUTIC TARGET

Although research into the effects of dysbiosis on the host abounds, the effects of the host on the microbiome are more limited. In a study done by Olivares and colleagues,[41] infants carrying the HLA-DQ2 haplotype influence the early microbiota composition, underlying the importance of host factors on microbial composition.

Genetic studies contribute to the concept recently described by Hooper and colleagues,[42] that the host exerts inside-out control over the microbiota, whereas the microbiota also exerts outside-in programming of host immunity and metabolism.

This cross-talk among the microbiota, host genetics, nutrition, immunity, and metabolism is initiated in infancy and continues throughout life. The window of opportunity to establish host immunity, and therefore inside-out control of the microbiome, depends on appropriate infant colonization through prenatal maternal exposures,[43] delivery mode,[6] breast-feeding,[44] and judicious use of antibiotics.

Although dysbiosis has been clearly associated with the development of autoimmunity, treatment strategies are still in their infancy. Ideally, in the future, treatments will be tailored to the cause of dysbiosis and will reflect knowledge of microbial-gut homeostasis. Once dysbiosis has already occurred, 2 main categories of treatment exist: (1) nutritional changes to encourage growth of normal endogenous microbes and (2) direct administration of live microorganisms.

To date, a gluten-free diet (GFD) is the only therapy for patients with CD; a GFD reduces symptoms and restores the well-being of the individual and heals the mucosal damage.[45] Several studies have compared the gut microbiota of patients with CD on and off a GFD and healthy controls. In patients with CD, even after following a GFD (for at least 2 years), the duodenal microbiota was not completely restored and showed a less abundant bacterial richness compared with healthy and untreated subjects, with a persistent imbalance of the ratio of potentially harmful/beneficial bacteria.[39] Species-specific analysis has shown that although E coli and Staphylococcus counts are restored after a GFD, Bifidobacterium counts remain lower in the feces of patients on a GFD compared with controls. A targeted study on Bifidobacterium composition from patients with CD on both a gluten-containing and a GFD and from healthy controls showed a correlation between the levels of total Bifidobacterium and Bifidobacterium longum species in the fecal and tissue samples. Moreover, a generalized reduction in these bacterial populations was found in patients with CD as compared with healthy children overall.[46]

Few studies have followed the same patients pre and post GFD to test the effect of gluten on the microbiome in the presence of CD. An Italian study showed that the Lactobacillus community was lower before than after a GFD and lower in patients with CD than in healthy controls. There was also a lower ratio of Bifidobacterium to Bacteroides and Enterobacteriaceae as compared with healthy controls.[45] Additional information comes from a study that evaluated the effect of a GFD on healthy subjects using fluorescence in situ hybridization and quantitative polymerase chain reaction.[34] In this study, it was noted that the GFD leads to a decrease in B longum, Clostridium lituseburense, Lactobacillus, and Faecalibacterium prausnitzii and an increase in Enterobacteriaceae and E coli strains. This was thought to be due to reduced production of proinflammatory and regulatory cytokines due to a generalized reduction in the total luminal bacterial load of the large intestine caused by the GFD. The main finding was that a GFD influenced gut microbial composition and immune activation (as measured by cytokine production) regardless of the presence of disease, and these effects were directly related to reduction in polysaccharide intake.

These studies show that a GFD only partially restores fecal microbiota balances in patients with CD. The reason is still unclear, although some suggest that genetic influences in those predisposed to CD affect the colonization of the microbiome, which persists despite a GFD; furthermore, because gluten has a prebiotic action, its absence in the GFD induces a different gut microbiota even in healthy individuals.[47]

In theory, probiotics represent a tempting fix to complex dysbiosis: identify the missing bacteria and replace them; in practice this has proved more difficult. Prebiotics are substances that induce the growth or activity of microorganisms (eg, bacteria and fungi) that contribute to the well-being of the host. Dietary prebiotics are typically nondigestible, fiber compounds that stimulate the growth of advantageous bacteria, although they do not target a specific bacterial group. Several foods are rich in prebiotics, including raw garlic, leeks, chicory root, and whole wheat (although not relevant to patients with CD). However, the ideal daily serving is not agreed on. Current research is ongoing as to the possibility of altering gluten-free products with prebiotics. Some early evidence has suggested that adding prebiotic inulin-type fructans to gluten-free breads can provide benefits for patients with CD, as these are ingredients that can increase calcium absorption and possibly other nutrients as well.[48]

Although prebiotics refer to the nutritional components found in food sources, probiotics are microorganisms that are believed to provide health benefits when consumed.[49] Live probiotic cultures are available in fermented dairy products and probiotic-fortified foods. Tablets, capsules, powders, and sachets also contain the bacteria in freeze-dried formulations. According to the Food and Agriculture Organization/World Health Organization, a probiotic is defined as a"live microorganism, which when administered in adequate amounts confers a health benefit on the host."[50] Probiotics have been found to be effective in some diseases, such as irritable bowel syndrome and pouchitis, but effects in other diseases, such as CD, have been less than conclusive. Some probiotics have been found to digest or alter gluten polypeptides. De Fallani and coworkers analyzed the potential role of the specific probiotic preparation VSL#3 (a cocktail of 8 strains that belong to the species *Bifidobacterium breve, B longum, B infantis, Lactobacillus plantarum, Lactobacillus acidophilus, Lactobacillus casei, Lactobacillus delbrueckii bulgaricus,* and *Streptococcus thermophiles*) in decreasing the toxic properties of wheat flour and found that VSL#3 was highly effective in hydrolyzing gliadin peptides. However, this ability was not noted with other probiotic preparations.[51] Specific *Lactobacillus* and bifidobacterial strains have been found to improve gut health. De Palma and collaborators[52] evaluated in vitro immunomodulatory properties of *Bifidobacterium bifidum* strain IATA-ES2 and *B longus* strain ATCC15707 versus *B fragilis* strain DSM2451, *E coli* strain CBL2, and *Shigella* spp on peripheral blood mononuclear cells under the effects of gliadin. This study found that *B bifidum* and *B longum* were able to induce lower levels of interleukin (IL)-12 and interferon (IFN)-γ production compared with *E coli* and *Shigella*. These bacteria were more likely to induce production of proinflammatory cytokines, which in turn contribute to development of disease. Lindfors and colleagues[53] found that *Bifidobacterium lactis* exerted a protective effect on epithelial cells against cellular damage induced by gliadin incubation. Recently, a study using a gliadin-induced enteropathy animal model was developed to observe whether *B longum* CECT 7347 could provide beneficial effects. The administration of this probiotic enhanced villus width and enterocyte height, which partially restored alterations in animals sensitized with IFN-γ and fed gliadin. It also decreased the levels of proinflammatory cytokines such as tumor necrosis factor-α (TNF-α) and increased levels of anti-inflammatory IL-10.[54]

Another study evaluating the effect of *B longum* CECT 7347 for 3 months in addition to a GFD in children newly diagnosed with CD showed a decrease in CD3 T cells, improving symptoms, and greater height percentile in those on a probiotic and GFD compared with those on the diet alone.[55]

Studies evaluating the role of probiotics and CD in humans are scarce. In a randomized, double-blind, placebo-controlled study, *B infantis* and its effects on gut permeability, occurrence of symptoms, and the presence of inflammatory cytokines in untreated patients with CD were evaluated. In this study, it was noted that probiotic administration was unable to modify gut barrier function; however, there was a marked improvement in digestion and a reduction in constipation. Abdominal pain and diarrheal symptom scores were also diminished, although not significantly. There was no difference in inflammatory markers.[56]

A study in children, studying the effect of *Bifidobacterium breve* BR03 and B632 on serum cytokine production, showed a decreased production of proinflammatory cytokine production after administration of probiotics compared with diet alone. The effect on proinflammatory cytokine TNF- α was seen only while receiving the probiotic, whereas anti-inflammatory cytokine IL-10 levels were undetectable throughout the study period, suggesting that continuous probiotic supplementation is necessary and intermittent administration does not affect microbial milieu.

Alternatively, members of the Firmicutes phylum, specifically lactobacilli, are thought to play a role in CD pathogenesis as well. A study identified a significant lack of *Lactobacillus* in symptom-free children with CD. Thus, the investigators isolated 5 different lactobacilli in the stool of healthy children, and proposed *Lactobacillus rhamnosus* and *Lactobacillus paracasei* as potential targets.[57]

Although preliminary research has suggested a possible role for probiotics in the treatment of CD, the relatively poor regulation of these supplements makes this treatment relatively hard to monitor. A study done testing 22 of the top-selling probiotics, labeled gluten-free, and using chromatography to check for presence of gluten showed that 12 (55%) of the 22 probiotics contained more than 20 ppm of gluten, the acceptable cutoff for labeling a food product as gluten-free.[58,59]

To date, the evidence regarding the use of probiotics in patients with CD is still insufficient to justify their use in clinical practice, and until the Food and Drug Administration places stricter regulations on these supplements, their use can be considered dangerous for patients with CD. The recent evidence that probiotics do not alter the fecal microbiome of healthy subjects adds to the question of their applicability to widespread use.[60]

SUMMARY

In recent years, as evidenced by the growing number of publications, an increasing amount of attention has been paid to the microbiome in health and disease. Although most publications on the microbiome in CD have been conducted using different models, study populations, and small sample sizes, most of the studies have seen differences in the populations of *Bifidobacterium* and *Lactobacillus* in the gut microbial concentrations of patients with CD. In addition, patients with CD seem to have an increased number of gram-negative bacteria, specifically *Proteobacteria.* In vitro data have suggested that dysbiosis in CD can lead to modification of the mucosal barrier, and persistent immune activation or sensitization to activation by gliadin causing clinical symptoms. Additional studies dissecting out the role of the microbiome in immune cell activation and T-cell priming will help further clarify the role of the microbiome in autoimmune disease pathogenesis and possibly the role of microbiome manipulation as treatment for CD.

As far as the GFD diet is concerned, it is currently the only accepted treatment for patients with CD. However, as evidenced by several studies, with regard to the microbiome, complete "normalization" is not achieved with this diet. In this setting is where probiotic therapy might be beneficial. Treatment with *Bifidobacterium* and/or *Lactobacillus* might be helpful in restoring altered gut microbiota and dampening immune activation, although further studies are needed to understand the dosing and proportion in which these bacteria need to be given for this to be achieved.

Finally, if considering the microbiome as a possible environmental activator for CD pathogenesis, it is possible to consider probiotics as a modulator of risk in those with high-risk factors, such as the DQ2 or DQ8 phenotype. In these subjects, probiotic administration might have a role in primary prevention; however, no study has been conducted using probiotics for this purpose, so much research needs to be done in this area before any conclusions can be made.

REFERENCES

1. Kau AL, Ahern PP, Griffin NW, et al. Human nutrition, the gut microbiome and the immune system. Nature 2011;474(7351):327–36.
2. Green PH, Cellier C. Celiac disease. N Engl J Med 2007;357(17):1731–43.
3. Sharma R, Young C, Neu J. Molecular modulation of intestinal epithelial barrier: contribution of microbiota. J Biomed Biotechnol 2010;2010:305879.
4. Kalliomaki M, Satokari R, Lahteenoja H, et al. Expression of microbiota, Toll-like receptors, and their regulators in the small intestinal mucosa in celiac disease. J Pediatr Gastroenterol Nutr 2012;54(6):727–32.
5. Stappenbeck TS, Hooper LV, Gordon JI. Developmental regulation of intestinal angiogenesis by indigenous microbes via Paneth cells. Proc Natl Acad Sci U S A 2002;99(24):15451–5.
6. Dominguez-Bello MG, Costello EK, Contreras M, et al. Delivery mode shapes the acquisition and structure of the initial microbiota across multiple body habitats in newborns. Proc Natl Acad Sci U S A 2010;107(26):11971–5.
7. Mackie RI, Sghir A, Gaskins HR. Developmental microbial ecology of the neonatal gastrointestinal tract. Am J Clin Nutr 1999;69(5):1035S–45S.
8. Jakobsson J, Stridsberg M, Zetterberg H, et al. Decreased cerebrospinal fluid secretogranin II concentrations in severe forms of bipolar disorder. J Psychiatry Neurosci 2013;38(4):E21–6.
9. Koenig JE, Spor A, Scalfone N, et al. Succession of microbial consortia in the developing infant gut microbiome. Proc Natl Acad Sci U S A 2011; 108(Suppl 1):4578–85.
10. Rautava S, Luoto R, Salminen S, et al. Microbial contact during pregnancy, intestinal colonization and human disease. Nat Rev Gastroenterol Hepatol 2012;9(10): 565–76.
11. Deplancke B, Gaskins HR. Microbial modulation of innate defense: goblet cells and the intestinal mucus layer. Am J Clin Nutr 2001;73(6):1131S–41S.
12. Everard A, Belzer C, Geurts L, et al. Cross-talk between *Akkermansia muciniphila* and intestinal epithelium controls diet-induced obesity. Proc Natl Acad Sci U S A 2013;110(22):9066–71.
13. Vaishnava S, Yamamoto M, Severson KM, et al. The antibacterial lectin RegIII-gamma promotes the spatial segregation of microbiota and host in the intestine. Science 2011;334(6053):255–8.
14. Gareau MG, Sherman PM, Walker WA. Probiotics and the gut microbiota in intestinal health and disease. Nat Rev Gastroenterol Hepatol 2010;7(9):503–14.
15. Fukuda S, Toh H, Hase K, et al. Bifidobacteria can protect from enteropathogenic infection through production of acetate. Nature 2011;469(7331):543–7.
16. Cebra JJ, Periwal SB, Lee G, et al. Development and maintenance of the gut-associated lymphoid tissue (GALT): the roles of enteric bacteria and viruses. Dev Immunol 1998;6(1–2):13–8.
17. Ibnou-Zekri N, Blum S, Schiffrin EJ, et al. Divergent patterns of colonization and immune response elicited from two intestinal *Lactobacillus* strains that display similar properties in vitro. Infect Immun 2003;71(1):428–36.
18. Peterson DA, McNulty NP, Guruge JL, et al. IgA response to symbiotic bacteria as a mediator of gut homeostasis. Cell Host Microbe 2007;2(5):328–39.

19. Sjogren YM, Tomicic S, Lundberg A, et al. Influence of early gut microbiota on the maturation of childhood mucosal and systemic immune responses. Clin Exp Allergy 2009;39(12):1842–51.

20. Bottcher MF, Haggstrom P, Bjorksten B, et al. Total and allergen-specific immunoglobulin A levels in saliva in relation to the development of allergy in infants up to 2 years of age. Clin Exp Allergy 2002;32(9):1293–8.

21. Elahi S, Ertelt JM, Kinder JM, et al. Immunosuppressive CD71+ erythroid cells compromise neonatal host defence against infection. Nature 2013;504(7478): 158–62.

22. Smith PM, Howitt MR, Panikov N, et al. The microbial metabolites, short-chain fatty acids, regulate colonic Treg cell homeostasis. Science 2013;341(6145):569–73.

23. Mazmanian SK, Liu CH, Tzianabos AO, et al. An immunomodulatory molecule of symbiotic bacteria directs maturation of the host immune system. Cell 2005; 122(1):107–18.

24. Maiuri L, Ciacci C, Ricciardelli I, et al. Association between innate response to gliadin and activation of pathogenic T cells in coeliac disease. Lancet 2003; 362(9377):30–7.

25. Ivanov II, Atarashi K, Manel N, et al. Induction of intestinal Th17 cells by segmented filamentous bacteria. Cell 2009;139(3):485–98.

26. Goto Y, Panea C, Nakato G, et al. Segmented filamentous bacteria antigens presented by intestinal dendritic cells drive mucosal Th17 cell differentiation. Immunity 2014;40(4):594–607.

27. Fernandez S, Molina IJ, Romero P, et al. Characterization of gliadin-specific Th17 cells from the mucosa of celiac disease patients. Am J Gastroenterol 2011; 106(3):528–38.

28. Decker E, Engelmann G, Findeisen A, et al. Cesarean delivery is associated with celiac disease but not inflammatory bowel disease in children. Pediatrics 2010; 125(6):e1433–40.

29. Sellitto M, Bai G, Serena G, et al. Proof of concept of microbiome-metabolome analysis and delayed gluten exposure on celiac disease autoimmunity in genetically at-risk infants. PLoS One 2012;7(3):e33387.

30. Cani PD, Possemiers S, Van de Wiele T, et al. Changes in gut microbiota control inflammation in obese mice through a mechanism involving GLP-2-driven improvement of gut permeability. Gut 2009;58(8):1091–103.

31. Cox LM, Yamanishi S, Sohn J, et al. Altering the intestinal microbiota during a critical developmental window has lasting metabolic consequences. Cell 2014; 158(4):705–21.

32. Kemppainen KM, Lynch KF, Liu E, et al. Factors that increase risk of celiac disease autoimmunity after a gastrointestinal infection in early life. Clin Gastroenterol Hepatol 2017;15(5):694–702 e5.

33. Bouziat R, Hinterleitner R, Brown JJ, et al. Reovirus infection triggers inflammatory responses to dietary antigens and development of celiac disease. Science 2017;356(6333):44–50.

34. De Palma G, Nadal I, Collado MC, et al. Effects of a gluten-free diet on gut microbiota and immune function in healthy adult human subjects. Br J Nutr 2009; 102(8):1154–60.

35. De Palma G, Nadal I, Medina M, et al. Intestinal dysbiosis and reduced immunoglobulin-coated bacteria associated with coeliac disease in children. BMC Microbiol 2010;10:63.

36. De Palma G, Capilla A, Nadal I, et al. Interplay between human leukocyte antigen genes and the microbial colonization process of the newborn intestine. Curr Issues Mol Biol 2010;12(1):1–10.

37. Nadal I, Santacruz A, Marcos A, et al. Shifts in clostridia, bacteroides and immunoglobulin-coating fecal bacteria associated with weight loss in obese adolescents. Int J Obes (Lond) 2009;33(7):758–67.

38. Nistal E, Caminero A, Herran AR, et al. Differences of small intestinal bacteria populations in adults and children with/without celiac disease: effect of age, gluten diet, and disease. Inflamm Bowel Dis 2012;18(4):649–56.

39. Collado MC, Donat E, Ribes-Koninckx C, et al. Specific duodenal and faecal bacterial groups associated with paediatric coeliac disease. J Clin Pathol 2009;62(3):264–9.

40. Noval Rivas M, Burton OT, Wise P, et al. A microbiota signature associated with experimental food allergy promotes allergic sensitization and anaphylaxis. J Allergy Clin Immunol 2013;131(1):201–12.

41. Olivares M, Neef A, Castillejo G, et al. The HLA-DQ2 genotype selects for early intestinal microbiota composition in infants at high risk of developing coeliac disease. Gut 2015;64(3):406–17.

42. Hooper LV, Littman DR, Macpherson AJ. Interactions between the microbiota and the immune system. Science 2012;336(6086):1268–73.

43. von Mutius E. Maternal farm exposure/ingestion of unpasteurized cow's milk and allergic disease. Curr Opin Gastroenterol 2012;28(6):570–6.

44. Perez PF, Dore J, Leclerc M, et al. Bacterial imprinting of the neonatal immune system: lessons from maternal cells? Pediatrics 2007;119(3):e724–32.

45. Guandalini S, Assiri A. Celiac disease: a review. JAMA Pediatr 2014;168(3):272–8.

46. Collado MC, Donat E, Ribes-Koninckx C, et al. Imbalances in faecal and duodenal Bifidobacterium species composition in active and non-active coeliac disease. BMC Microbiol 2008;8:232.

47. Di Cagno R, Rizzello CG, Gagliardi F, et al. Different fecal microbiotas and volatile organic compounds in treated and untreated children with celiac disease. Appl Environ Microbiol 2009;75(12):3963–71.

48. Capriles VD, Areas JA. Effects of prebiotic inulin-type fructans on structure, quality, sensory acceptance and glycemic response of gluten-free breads. Food Funct 2013;4(1):104–10.

49. Rijkers GT, de Vos WM, Brummer RJ, et al. Health benefits and health claims of probiotics: bridging science and marketing. Br J Nutr 2011;106(9):1291–6.

50. Food and Agriculture Organization of the United Nations WHO. Guidelines for the evaluation of probiotics in food. Geneva (Switzerland): World Health Organization; 2002.

51. Fallani M, Young D, Scott J, et al. Intestinal microbiota of 6-week-old infants across Europe: geographic influence beyond delivery mode, breast-feeding, and antibiotics. J Pediatr Gastroenterol Nutr 2010;51(1):77–84.

52. De Palma G, Cinova J, Stepankova R, et al. Pivotal advance: Bifidobacteria and Gram-negative bacteria differentially influence immune responses in the proinflammatory milieu of celiac disease. J Leukoc Biol 2010;87(5):765–78.

53. Lindfors K, Blomqvist T, Juuti-Uusitalo K, et al. Live probiotic Bifidobacterium lactis bacteria inhibit the toxic effects induced by wheat gliadin in epithelial cell culture. Clin Exp Immunol 2008;152(3):552–8.

54. Laparra JM, Olivares M, Gallina O, et al. *Bifidobacterium longum* CECT 7347 modulates immune responses in a gliadin-induced enteropathy animal model. PLoS One 2012;7(2):e30744.
55. Olivares M, Castillejo G, Varea V, et al. Double-blind, randomised, placebo-controlled intervention trial to evaluate the effects of *Bifidobacterium longum* CECT 7347 in children with newly diagnosed coeliac disease. Br J Nutr 2014; 112(1):30–40.
56. Smecuol E, Hwang HJ, Sugai E, et al. Exploratory, randomized, double-blind, placebo-controlled study on the effects of *Bifidobacterium infantis natren* life start strain super strain in active celiac disease. J Clin Gastroenterol 2013;47(2): 139–47.
57. Lorenzo Pisarello MJ, Vintini EO, Gonzalez SN, et al. Decrease in lactobacilli in the intestinal microbiota of celiac children with a gluten-free diet, and selection of potentially probiotic strains. Can J Microbiol 2015;61(1):32–7.
58. Nazareth S, Lebwohl B, Voyksner JS, et al. Widespread contamination of probiotics with gluten, detected by liquid chromatography-mass spectrometry. Gastroenterology 2015;148:S28.
59. Vanderpool C, Yan F, Polk DB. Mechanisms of probiotic action: implications for therapeutic applications in inflammatory bowel diseases. Inflamm Bowel Dis 2008;14(11):1585–96.
60. Kristensen NB, Bryrup T, Allin KH, et al. Alterations in fecal microbiota composition by probiotic supplementation in healthy adults: a systematic review of randomized controlled trials. Genome Med 2016;8(1):52.

Follow-up of Celiac Disease

Steffen Husby, MD, PhD[a],*, Julio C. Bai, MD[b]

KEYWORDS

- Follow-up • Gluten-free diet • Mucosal healing • Serology • Adherence • Adults
- Children and adolescents

KEY POINTS

- Much discussion in celiac disease has centered on the diagnosis; in contrast, management and follow-up have had a lesser interest in celiac disease.
- Follow-up is tightly related to adherence to the gluten-free diet (GFD).
- A GFD normally leads to significant improvement in symptoms, normalization of biochemical measures, and increase in quality of life in patients reporting symptoms at baseline, but does not always result in optimal management.

IMPORTANCE OF FOLLOW-UP

Much discussion in celiac disease (CD) has centered on the diagnosis; consequently management and follow-up have had a less pertinent role, even though CD in the adult population is accompanied by persistent symptoms and mucosal changes in 20% to 40% of cases,[1] much less in children and adolescents (**Box 1**). In this article, the perspective of both the pediatric and adult gastroenterologist will be given as to management and follow-up. Follow-up is tightly related to adherence to the main treatment, the gluten-free diet (GFD).

WHY CELIAC DISEASE PATIENTS SHOULD BE FOLLOWED-UP?

Currently, the only effective treatment for CD is complete avoidance of gluten from the diet. A GFD can lead to significant improvement in symptoms, normalization of biochemical measures, and increase in quality of life in patients reporting symptoms at baseline. Because CD is an inflammatory condition that affects multiple organ systems, there are multiple pieces of evidence, although weak, that lifelong treatment may reduce the risk of malignant and nonmalignant complications that may implicate

Disclosure: Steffen Husby has participated in advisory board for Inova, has received honorarium as a speaker from Thermo-Fisher, and unrestricted research grants from Thermo-Fisher and Takeda.

[a] Hans Christian Andersen Children's Hospital, Odense University Hospital, Kløvervaenget 23C, Odense C, DK-5000, Denmark; [b] Hospital de Gastroenterología Dr. C. Bonorino Udaondo, Av. Caseros 2061, Buenos Aires 1236, Argentina
* Corresponding author.
E-mail address: Steffen.husby@rsyd.dk

Gastroenterol Clin N Am 48 (2019) 127–136
https://doi.org/10.1016/j.gtc.2018.09.009
0889-8553/19/© 2018 Elsevier Inc. All rights reserved.

gastro.theclinics.com

Box 1
The NICE guidelines, from the United Kingdom, recommend a yearly review for all people with celiac disease

- Measuring weight and height
- Review of symptoms
- Considering the need for assessment of diet and adherence to the gluten-free diet
- Considering the need for specialist dietetic and nutritional advice
- Considering the need for referral to a general physician or consultant to address any concerns about possible complications or comorbidities.

Data from Ludvigsson JF, Bai JC, Biagi F, et al. Diagnosis and management of adult coeliac disease: guidelines from the British Society of Gastroenterology. Gut 2014;63(8):1210–28.

---

increased mortality.[2] A GFD has an intrinsic degree of difficulty, which relates to the following dietary measurements in general. In the present context, studies have reported low patient satisfaction for treatment, high costs for the GFD, and even continued symptoms and histologic signs of intestinal damage. As a result, the GFD does not always result in optimal management.

Although it is generally accepted that all wheat (gluten), rye (secalin), and barley (hordein) products must be strictly avoided in the GFD, the relationship between the quantity of gluten ingested and the development of symptoms and histologic abnormalities is not clearly defined and the exact amount of gluten that people with CD can tolerate on a daily basis without suffering any deleterious effects has not been fully established; in other terms, it is necessary to understand how strict a GFD needs to be.

Former studies have focused on the effect of disease on specific long-term clinical consequences such as mortality, bone damage, neurologic complications, autoimmune associations etc. Specifically, the possibility has been discussed whether on the one hand these complications could be modified by the GF and on the other hand how important the degree of adherence to the diet is in order to obtain favorable outcomes. An early study from Italy suggested a notably higher mortality (5 times greater than expected) in patients not adhering or partially adhering to the GFD.[3] Most studies assessing outcome of untreated adult patients were performed on symptomatic cases. In contrast, very few studies assessed the natural history of undiagnosed adults. Several studies have shown that patients, asymptomatic or oligosymptomatic at the time of diagnosis, have impaired bone densities or may have affected quality of life.[4,5] Very recently, a case-control study of adults without prior diagnosis of CD has shown that this population before diagnosis is more likely to develop osteoporosis, dermatitis herpetiformis, chronic fatigue, thyroiditis, or autoimmune diseases in general.[6]

WHAT IS APPROPRIATE FOR BEING CONSIDERED AS A GLUTEN-FREE DIET?

Concerns remain about the daily adherence to the GFD that could be involuntary or intentional and is an issue in adult patients.[7] As little as 50 mg of gluten, an amount present in a few crumbs of bread or a small piece of pasta, or traces of contamination, can produce symptoms and/or increase enteropathy in patients with asymptomatic CD, and maintaining a lifelong GFD is necessary for all patients. However, an accurate and cost-effective tool to monitor healing that avoids the need for regular endoscopies in symptomatic patients remains an unmet need.

GENERAL PRACTITIONER OR GASTROENTEROLOGIST?

In children, follow-up by the pediatric gastroenterologist is a natural consequence of the organization in pediatric subspecialties. In adults, the gastroenterologist may be responsible for the diagnosis including endoscopy, and the follow-up is often handed over to the GP, who knows the patient at a broad scale. In practice, the follow-up may then be offered at yearly intervals or at complications, when the management may be returned to the gastroenterologist. However, follow-up is frequently not performed, especially in young adults, perhaps the group with the greatest need.[8,9]

ROLE OF THE DIETICIAN

The management and follow-up of patients with CD is preferentially a team work.[10] Dietary counseling is an important area, which is well taken care of by an expert dietician. Patient adherence extremely depends on age and the general attitude of the patient, who may resort to dietary digressions during puberty/adolescence and less so after that age. The advice of the dietician may be the best instrument in maintaining the patient adherence. The competence of the patient increases after the first few years of GFD and the adult patient in general feels adequately competent, whereas the child and adolescent may feel more insecure and concerned.[11] Cereals containing gluten are rich in dietary fibers, iron, and multiple B vitamins, so the risk of low intake of dietary fiber, B vitamins, and iron in the GFD needs to be taken care of in the dietetic consultation.[12,13] In most, but not all, patients, oats that are uncontaminated may be tolerated and introduced in the GFD after clinical and serologic stabilization has been achieved.[14,15]

CHILDREN AND ADOLESCENTS

The recommended yearly review of those with celiac disease after remission has been obtained, including children and adolescents. Preferentially, the follow-up concentrates not only on energy, growth, and vitamin insufficiencies but as well on general development and coping strategies. Recent publications show that at the time of disease diagnosis the patient may have deficiencies in calcium, iron, vitamin B12, and folate.[16] However, these deficiencies disappeared at the first and following reviews. No hypocalcemia or thyroid dysfunction was found. Vitamin D insufficiency was an exception, and the levels equaled those of healthy children at the same age, reflecting the current discussion of sufficient values of vitamin D.[17] Thus, the follow-up should be problem oriented based on symptoms and signs, rather than a routine screening of malabsorption parameters.

Still, in children and adolescents a satisfactory increase in weight and height is an essential marker of the success of the GFD. In general, young people/teenagers are less satisfied with the impact of CD on their lives[18] and even less adherent to a GFD than adults.[19] Whether the diagnosis of CD is based on symptoms or obtained by screening seemingly does not influence children's and adolescents' later adherence to GFD.[20] As stated earlier, therapy-resistant CD is of rare occurrence in children.[21] However, children who are lost to follow-up more frequently are nonadherent to GFD and are antibody positive, showing that follow-up is not unimportant.[22]

Recently, the option to make the diagnosis of CD in children and adolescents without a duodenal biopsy has been introduced in European guidelines.[23] The utility of this option is based on the finding that high positive IgA transglutaminase antibodies (TG2-IgA) as a diagnostic tool was shown to correlate to mucosal changes corresponding to Marsh II or III.[24] The high positive TG2-IgA should be demonstrated in 2 separate blood samples and accompanied by a positive endomysial antibody (EMA) test. The no-biopsy diagnostic approach includes a reduction of symptoms and antibody levels after the introduction of GFD. Gastroscopy and duodenal biopsies in children and adolescents require general anesthesia, which makes the procedure more cumbersome, and is avoided by the no-biopsy approach. Concerns have been raised because the biopsy and the gastroscopy will assure that other diagnoses are not overlooked.[25] However, this seems not to be a problem in clinical practice.[26] In children and adolescents a follow-up biopsy is only done when remission has not been achieved, because clinical remission is by far the rule and lack of response to a GFD the exception.

A key issue in the follow-up is the usefulness of serology, whether a decline and subsequent normalization of antibody levels is sufficient evidence for proper management.[27,28] Limited usefulness of serology has been reported in childhood CD but probably with a better performance in the long term.[29] In a recent meta-analysis the positive predictive value and the sensitivity of positive TG2-IgA determination was fairly low for adults, but higher (0.70) for children. The negative predictive value of serology in adult patients on a gluten-free diet for 1 year or more was reasonably high and 0.87 for children.[30] This pattern was also seen for EMA antibodies, where the positive predictive value and the sensitivity was low in adults (0.39) and high in children (0.78), whereas the negative predictive value and the specificity was reasonably high for adults as well as for children, 0.93 and 0.78, respectively. A refinement of the TG2-IgA determination, using the detectable levels below the upper normal limit has been shown to add the identification of adult CD patients with mucosal healing[31] and could be of use also in children and adolescents. It may be concluded that the usefulness of serology at follow-up is uncertain; however, CD diagnosed in children and adolescents mostly leads to mucosal healing. The process of transition from childhood into adulthood is in general a time that calls for tolerance as well as persistence from the caregiver and when most patients experience a period of uncertainty.[32]

FOLLOW-UP IN ADULTS

Adults are more independent individuals who usually challenge professional decisions and recommendations. Social and professional activities as their access to gluten-free products often are relevant contexts framing the degree of adherence to the GFD. As commented before, adults on a GFD can have an asymptomatic clinical course but a proportion of cases can experience symptom relapse (either gastrointestinal or extraintestinal symptoms) or may be persistently symptomatic since diagnosis, a clinical characteristic that is different to treated children with CD.[33] The proportion of cases in each group is variable among studies. Persistence of symptoms has many potential causes (see later discussion).

A thorough clinical evaluation is a relevant part of the follow-up of patients. In such an event, checking symptoms and doing general laboratory tests (eg, full blood count, serum iron, vitamin B_{12}, folic acid, calcium, vitamin D serum status) and CD serology tests are the most recommended tests to be performed at any interview. A bone mineral density scan (DXA scanning) can be performed at baseline (diagnosis) to provide measure of bone mass. Vitamin or mineral supplementation is required in patients with deficits or in cases with bone derangement. In cases with osteopenia or osteoporosis, the strict GFD is the best treatment of the bone affection. Long-term improvement in bone density and bone microstructure is the best that can be obtained.[32] If baseline bone density is normal, a new determination should only be produced for women at the time of menopause.

Vaccination against pneumococci, *Haemophilus influenza* and meningococci are strongly recommended.[34] The patient should be helped to join support groups with acknowledged experience in CD. In this context, levels of adherence to gluten-free diet are associated with membership of advocacy groups and regular dietetic follow-up. If necessary and/or requested, a psychologist consultation should be offered.[35] As it is in childhood CD, serology is the cornerstone in the diagnostic workup of adults. As mentioned earlier, immunoglobulin A (IgA) antibodies to tissue transglutaminase is a central diagnostic tests for active CD, even though the evidence base of the specific antibody determinations is weak.[36,37] Decreasing concentrations of antibodies indicate an effective GFD, as has been shown by a prospective study of kinetics of CD-specific antibodies.[38] Positive concentrations of antibodies may be regarded as indicators of improvement; however, they have limited sensitivity to define complete adherence. Once the antibodies have normalized, a subsequent increase in level is considered a good indicator of gluten ingestion.[28] In contrast, serologic tests cannot detect minor dietary indiscretions (traces) or intermittent consumption and, therefore, normal titers are insensitive for ongoing gluten exposure or enteropathy.

For many, the ultimate measure of adherence is the demonstration of intestinal healing, but this may not occur even in patients with strict gluten avoidance.[1] The need for repeated duodenal biopsies to evaluate healing and to assess adherence to a GFD is controversial. Although this approach is frequently used in practice, it is not clear whether it is necessary for patients who respond to the GFD clinically and have decreasing or negative celiac antibody levels. Complete healing of the intestinal mucosa is also often slow or incomplete, for further discussion see below. Intestinal biopsies should be considered mandatory in patients with persistent symptoms despite consistent evidence of a strict GFD.[4] Recently published recommendations for procuration, processing, and analysis of diagnostic biopsy of CD in adult patients are available. However, these recommendations do not fit within the theoretic necessity of follow-up biopsies.[35] Several questions may be asked: how to deal with the potential patchy damage of the duodenum. How do biopsies represent the small bowel enteropathy? How to report damage, by using Marsh classification, including intraepithelial count as well as villus/crypt ratio? How frequently should biopsies be taken if complete recovery is not produced? How to proceed after a set of samples with recovered histology? Does healing exclude further relapse? Although some studies have shown that persistent damage can be associated with clinical deterioration and even increased mortality, these observations are not shared by others.[39,40] In this complex context, follow-up biopsies do not seem to be required except for patients who are persistently symptomatic despite no evidence of dietary indiscretions and/or with normal serology. Thus, decision to follow-up treated patients is mostly based on expert consensus.

Consultation with a registered dietitian is considered as an essential step to obtain the best results for accessing to the therapeutic goals. Although there is no gold standard for assessing dietary adherence, there is a general consensus that this assessment in the multidisciplinary evaluation is part of the best follow-up strategy. Ideally, consultations to an expert dietitian should be produced every 3 to 6 months until clinical stabilization, then every 1 to 2 years. This is particularly important in women of child-bearing age and during pregnancy. The role of the dietician is crucial (**Box 2**). Patients who are unable to adhere to the diet may require support with psychological counseling.

Box 2
Tasks for the dietician at follow-up

1. Assess nutritional status

2. Identify macronutrient and/or micronutrient detect, deficiencies, and/or excesses

3. Analyze eating habits and potential factors affecting access to the diet

4. Provide information and initiate the gluten-free diet

5. Provide dietary education

6. Monitor and evaluate dietary compliance and reinforce alimentary counseling

---

MUCOSAL HEALING

Mucosal healing in adults is based on the assessment of follow-up duodenal biopsies. Some investigators have suggested that it is important to perform a duodenal biopsy to assess the recovery of intestinal mucosa and to exclude refractory CD and malignancies. Although a normal follow-up histology is strongly informative about the degree of adherence to the GFD, this may not occur even in patients with strict gluten avoidance. The need for repeated duodenal biopsies to evaluate healing and assess adherence to a GFD is still a controversial matter. Although the repeat biopsy approach is frequently used in practice, it is not clear whether it is necessary for patients who clinically respond to the GFD and have decreasing or negative auto-antibody levels. A series of findings from recently published retrospective studies are in favor of biopsy follow-up.[41] However, the timing and localization for sampling, reporting results (whether semiquantitative—Marsh's modified staging—or quantitative morphology), limits of the number of repeated endoscopies and biopsy procuration, and cost of such strategies have not been established. A more conservative follow-up suggests to reserve biopsy for those cases with persistent symptoms despite a negative (normal) CD-specific serology and no evidence of dietary indiscretions (**Fig. 1**). Obviously, both strategies aim to serve the best interest of patients and a cost-effective analysis is lacking. In the case of suspicion of refractory celiac disease (RCD I and II) an appropriate algorithm is required (which is not motif of analysis for this review).

REAL-TIME ASSESSMENT OF ADHERENCE

Recently, new quantitative ELISA (for stool) and quantitative immunocromatography (for urine) have emerged as tools that determine the consumption of gluten by assessing excretion of gluten immunogenic peptides (GIP).[42,43] These tests are based on the detection of GIP in stool and urine by monoclonal antibodies (anti-33 mer α-gliadin peptide G12). Previous studies have shown that a positive result constitutes specific evidence of dietary indiscretions. In addition to these, point-of-care tests (both for stool and urine) have been developed to simplify their use by patients at home or by physicians at the office. Notably, GIP tests for stool and urine can detect gluten consumption in symptomatic and asymptomatic patients unaware of dietary indiscretions. However, their utility in real life is still unclear. Likely, refining their sensitivity for detecting gluten consumption, which is estimated greater than 50 mg of gluten/d for stool tests and above 400 g/d for urine tests, seems necessary.[42] In any way, these newly developed laboratory-based, home-based, or office-based tests provide a sensitive and specific option for monitoring real-time dietary adherence to the GFD.

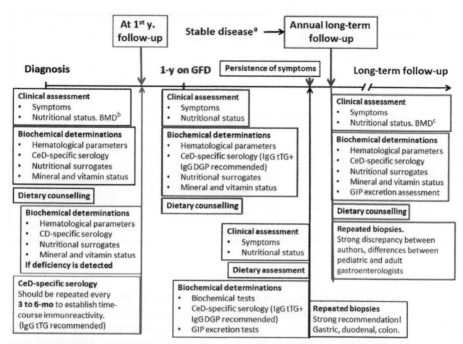

Fig. 1. Routine assessment for follow-up of patients with CD. [a] Stable disease: patients on a gluten-free diet without symptoms, signs, and/or abnormal biochemical tests (including CD-specific serology). [b] BMD: bone mineral density at diagnosis. [c] BMD at follow-up: only for cases with abnormal BMD (severe osteopenia or osteoporosis) at diagnosis or for patients not adherent to the gluten-free diet.

INTERVAL FOR ASSESSMENT OF ADULT PATIENTS AFTER DIAGNOSIS

It seems cost-effective to have knowledge of compliance with the GFD according to the time after diagnosis and the clinical status of patients. There is evidence suggesting that assessment should not be different for asymptomatic and symptomatic patients at follow-up. However, decisions are, in general, based on expert opinions. Guidelines suggest that patients should be controlled by a multidisciplinary team each 3 to 6 months from diagnosis to stabilization. After substantial improvement has been obtained, annual evaluation is recommended.

NONRESPONSIVE CELIAC DISEASE

Nonresponsive CD is considered when patients have persistent symptoms or mucosal damage is present despite a seemingly adequate GFD. Persistence of symptoms is frequently caused by continued ingestion of gluten. A common difficulty with the GFD is cross-contamination and the presence of unexpected gluten in processed food items and/or medicines. Gluten is used widely in processed food products and thus may be a hidden ingredient, so it is prudent for patients to routinely check the ingredient list before purchasing any product. If the response to the GFD is suboptimal, intentional, or inadvertent, ingestion of gluten should be considered. In these cases, persistence of positive serology may identify major and continued lapses in dietary adherence. Causes of persistence of symptoms in patients with CD are listed in **Box 3**.

Box 3
Causes of persistent symptoms in adults

1. Inadvertent or intentional gluten ingestion

2. Irritable bowel syndrome

3. Wrong diagnosis

4. Primary or secondary lactose intolerance

5. Food allergies

6. Pancreatic insufficiency

7. Microscopic colitis

8. Bacterial overgrowth

9. Refractory CD type I and II

10. Others

SUMMARY

Follow-up in CD is mutually important for children and adults. The timing of follow-up in uncomplicated cases usually can be restricted to a yearly basis. The contents of the follow-up may be blood tests including celiac antibodies, hematology, and a limited number of routine tests. A follow-up biopsy with the possibility to assess mucosal healing is the center of current discussion.

REFERENCES

1. Rubio-Tapia A, Rahim MW, See JA, et al. Mucosal recovery and mortality in adults with celiac disease after treatment with a gluten-free diet. Am J Gastroenterol 2010;105(6):1412–20.

2. Ludvigsson JF. Mortality and malignancy in celiac disease. Gastrointest Endosc Clin N Am 2012;22(4):705–22.

3. Corrao G, Corazza GR, Bagnardi V, et al, Club del Tenue Study Group. Mortality in patients with coeliac disease and their relatives: a cohort study. Lancet 2001; 358(9279):356–61.

4. Zanchetta MB, Costa AF, Longobardi V, et al. Improved bone microarchitecture in patients with celiac disease after 3 years on a gluten-free diet. Clin Gastroenterol Hepatol 2018;16(5):774–5.

5. Nachman F, Mauriño E, Vázquez H, et al. Quality of life in celiac disease patients: prospective analysis on the importance of clinical severity at diagnosis and the impact of treatment. Dig Liver Dis 2009;41(1):15–25.

6. Hujoel IA, Van Dyke CT, Brantner T, et al. Natural history and clinical detection of undiagnosed coeliac disease in a North American community. Aliment Pharmacol Ther 2018;47(10):1358–66.

7. Mahadev S, Murray JA, Wu TT, et al. Factors associated with villus atrophy in symptomatic coeliac disease patients on a gluten-free diet. Aliment Pharmacol Ther 2017;45(8):1084–93.

8. Hall NJ, Rubin G, Charnock A. Systematic review: adherence to a gluten-free diet in adult patients with coeliac disease. Aliment Pharmacol Ther 2009;30(4): 315–30.

9. Cohen ME, Jaffe A, Strauch CB, et al. Determinants of follow-up care for patients with celiac disease. J Clin Gastroenterol 2018;52(9):784–8.
10. See JA, Kaukinen K, Makharia GK, et al. Practical insights into gluten-free diets. Nat Rev Gastroenterol Hepatol 2015;12(10):580–91.
11. Kipp T, Skjerning H, Husby S. The large majority of coeliac children, adolescents and adults have a high degree of perceived dietary competence. Abstract presented at the Annual Meeting of ESPGHAN. May, 2018.
12. Ciacci C, Cirillo M, Cavallaro R, et al. Long-term follow-up of celiac adults on gluten-free diet: prevalence and correlates of intestinal damage. Digestion 2002;66(3):178–85.
13. Kinsey L, Burden ST, Bannerman E. A dietary survey to determine if patients with coeliac disease are meeting current healthy eating guidelines and how their diet compares to that of the British general population. Eur J Clin Nutr 2008;62(11): 1333–42.
14. Högberg L, Laurin P, Fälth-Magnusson K, et al. Oats to children with newly diagnosed coeliac disease: a randomised double blind study. Gut 2004;53(5): 649–54.
15. Lionetti E, Gatti S, Galeazzi T, et al. Safety of oats in children with celiac disease: a double-blind, randomized, placebo-controlled trial. J Pediatr 2018;194: 116–22.e2.
16. Wessels MM, van Veen II, Vriezinga SL, et al. Complementary serologic investigations in children with celiac disease is unnecessary during follow-up. J Pediatr 2016;169:55–60.
17. Deora V, Aylward N, Sokoro A, et al. Serum vitamins and minerals at diagnosis and follow-up in children with celiac disease. J Pediatr Gastroenterol Nutr 2017;65(2):185–9.
18. Ukkola A1, Mäki M, Kurppa K, et al. Patients' experiences and perceptions of living with coeliac disease - implications for optimizing care. J Gastrointestin Liver Dis 2012;21(1):17–22.
19. Kurppa K1, Lauronen O, Collin P, et al. Factors associated with dietary adherence in celiac disease: a nationwide study. Digestion 2012;86(4):309–14.
20. Kivelä L, Kaukinen K, Huhtala H, et al. At-risk screened children with celiac disease are comparable in disease severity and dietary adherence to those found because of clinical suspicion: a large cohort study. J Pediatr 2017;183: 115–21.e2.
21. Reilly NR1, Aguilar K, Hassid BG, et al. Celiac disease in normal-weight and overweight children: clinical features and growth outcomes following a gluten-free diet. J Pediatr Gastroenterol Nutr 2011;53(5):528–31.
22. Barnea L, Mozer-Glassberg Y, Hojsak I, et al. Pediatric celiac disease patients who are lost to follow-up have a poorly controlled disease. Digestion 2014; 90(4):248–53.
23. Husby S, Koletzko S, Korponay-Szabó IR, et al, ESPGHAN Working Group on Coeliac Disease Diagnosis, ESPGHAN Gastroenterology Committee. European Society for Pediatric Gastroenterology, Hepatology, and Nutrition guidelines for the diagnosis of coeliac disease. J Pediatr Gastroenterol Nutr 2012;54(1):136–60.
24. Giersiepen K, Lelgemann M, Stuhldreher N, et al, ESPGHAN Working Group on Coeliac Disease Diagnosis. Accuracy of diagnostic antibody tests for coeliac disease in children: summary of an evidence report. J Pediatr Gastroenterol Nutr 2012;54(2):229–41.
25. Guandalini S, Newland C. Can we really skip the biopsy in diagnosing symptomatic celiac children? J Pediatr Gastroenterol Nutr 2013;57:e24.

26. Husby S, Koletzko S, Korponay-Zsabo. Author's response. J Pediatr Gastroenterol Nutr 2013;57:e24.
27. Nachman F, del Campo MP, González A, et al. Long-term deterioration of quality of life in adult patients with celiac disease is associated with treatment noncompliance. Dig Liver Dis 2010;42(10):685–91.
28. Nachman F, Sugai E, Vázquez H, et al. Serological tests for celiac disease as indicators of long-term compliance with the gluten-free diet. Eur J Gastroenterol Hepatol 2011;23(6):473–80.
29. Vécsei E, Steinwendner S, Kogler H, et al. Follow-up of pediatric celiac disease: value of antibodies in predicting mucosal healing, a prospective cohort study. BMC Gastroenterol 2014;14:28.
30. Silvester JA, Kurada S, Szwajcer A, et al. Tests for serum transglutaminase and endomysial antibodies do not detect most patients with celiac disease and persistent villus atrophy on gluten-free diets: a meta-analysis. Gastroenterology 2017;153(3):689–701.e1.
31. Fang H, King KS, Larson JJ, et al. Undetectable negative tissue transglutaminase IgA antibodies predict mucosal healing in treated coeliac disease patients. Aliment Pharmacol Ther 2017;46(7):681–7.
32. Ludvigsson JF, Agreus L, Ciacci C, et al. Transition from childhood to adulthood in coeliac disease: the Prague consensus report. Gut 2016;65(8):1242–51.
33. Bai JC, Ciacci C. World Gastroenterology Organisation global guidelines: celiac disease February 2017. J Clin Gastroenterol 2017;51(9):755–68.
34. Kelly CP, Bai JC, Liu E, et al. Advances in diagnosis and management of celiac disease. Gastroenterology 2015;148(6):1175–86.
35. Ludvigsson JF, Bai JC, Biagi F, et al, Authors of the BSG Coeliac Disease Guidelines Development Group, British Society of Gastroenterology. Diagnosis and management of adult coeliac disease: guidelines from the British Society of Gastroenterology. Gut 2014;63(8):1210–28.
36. NICE:Coeliac disease: recognition, assessment and management, NICE guideline [NG20]. 2015. Available at: https://www.nice.org.uk/guidance/ng20.
37. Sugai E, Nachman F, Váquez H, et al. Dynamics of celiac disease-specific serology after initiation of a gluten-free diet and use in the assessment of compliance with treatment. Dig Liver Dis 2010;42:352–8.
38. Lebwohl B, Michaëlsson K, Green PH, et al. Persistent mucosal damage and risk of fracture in celiac disease. J Clin Endocrinol Metab 2014;99:609–16.
39. Lebwohl B, Granath F, Ekbom A, et al. Mucosal healing and risk for lymphoproliferative malignancy in celiac disease: a population-based cohort study. Ann Intern Med 2013;159:169–75.
40. Comino I, Real A, Vivas S, et al. Monitoring of gluten-free diet compliance in celiac patients by assessment of gliadin 33-mer equivalent epitopes in feces. Am J Clin Nutr 2012;95:670–7.
41. Lebwohl B, Granath F, Ekbom A, et al. Mucosal healing and mortality in coeliac disease. Aliment Pharmacol Ther 2013;37:332–9.
42. Moreno ML, Cebolla Á, Muñoz-Suano A, et al. Detection of gluten immunogenic peptides in the urine of patients with coeliac disease reveals transgressions in the gluten-free diet and incomplete mucosal healing. Gut 2017;66:250–7.
43. Syage JA, Kelly CP, Dickason MA, et al. Determination of gluten consumption in celiac disease patients on a gluten-free diet. Am J Clin Nutr 2018;107:201–7.

Refractory Celiac Disease

Georgia Malamut, MD, PhD[a,b,c],*, Christophe Cellier, MD, PhD[a,b,c]

KEYWORDS

- Refractory celiac disease • Phenotype of intraepithelial lymphocytes
- Cytokine IL-15 • Enteropathy-associated T-cell lymphoma

KEY POINTS

- Refractory celiac disease (RCD) refers to 2 distinct entities according to the normal (RCDI) or abnormal (RCDII) phenotype of intestinal intraepithelial lymphocytes.
- Diagnosis requires specialized small bowel investigations (enteroscopy, small bowel imaging) and techniques (immunohistochemistry, molecular analysis, flow cytometry).
- Prognosis of RCDII is worse than RCDI because of more severe malnutrition and an elevated risk of overt lymphoma.
- Therapeutic arsenal is currently mainly based on open capsule budesonide waiting for efficient targeted therapy.

INTRODUCTION

Treatment of celiac disease (CD) relies on a lifelong strict gluten-free diet that allows clinical and histologic recovery after 1 year of gluten-free diet and prevents long-term complications, such as osteopenia,[1] onset of other autoimmune disease,[2] and malignancies.[3] Yet, systematic follow-up of biopsies has revealed that histologic recovery does not occur in all patients. Notably, one recent population-based study led in 7648 patients with celiac disease in Sweden showed persistent villus atrophy in 43% of cases with an increased risk in older patients (up to 56% vs 17% in children diagnosed after 2000).[4] The similar rates of persistent villus atrophy among patients with CD biopsied 1 to 2 years and 2 to 5 years after diagnosis further argued against mucosal healing after 2 years.[4] Importantly, lack of mucosal healing has been associated with a risk of complications; it is notably a risk factor for fractures[5] and for the development of lymphomas.[6] Most cases of resistance to gluten-free diet (GFD) and persistence of villus atrophy are due to bad observance.[7] Nevertheless, a small subgroup of patients with CD may be primarily or secondarily resistant to a GFD due to an authentic refractory CD (RCD) with persistent symptoms of malabsorption

[a] Paris Descartes University, 15 rue de l'Ecole de Médecine, Paris 75006, France; [b] Gastroenterology Department, Hôpital Européen Georges Pompidou, APHP, 20 rue Leblanc, Paris 75015, France; [c] UMR1163 Institute Imagine, 24 Boulevard du Montparnasse, Paris 75015, France
* Corresponding author. Hôpital Européen Georges Pompidou, 20 rue Leblanc, Paris 75015, France.
E-mail address: georgia.malamut@aphp.fr

Gastroenterol Clin N Am 48 (2019) 137–144
https://doi.org/10.1016/j.gtc.2018.09.010
0889-8553/19/© 2018 Elsevier Inc. All rights reserved.

gastro.theclinics.com

and intestinal villus atrophy despite a strict GFD. Diagnosis of this condition is made after exclusion of other intestinal diseases with villus atrophy such as autoimmune enteropathy, tropical sprue, common variable immunodeficiency or drug-induced enteropathy.[8–11]

Frequency of RCD remains unknown. A North American referral center suggests a cumulative incidence of 1.5% for both RCDI and RCDII among patients with CD diagnosed in this center.[12] In the Derby cohort, J. West and G. Holmes report approximately 0.7% of patients with RCD with ulcerative jejunitis in series of 713 patients with CD.[13] Respective proportion of both types of RCD is also undefined with apparently a higher frequency of RCDI than RCDII in US[14] studies in contrast with European studies.[15–18]

DIAGNOSIS

Diagnosis of RCD relies on persisting malabsorption and villus atrophy after 1 to 2 years of strict GFD. Compliance of GFD can be ascertained by a dietician and dosage of serum celiac antibodies immunoglobulin (Ig)A and IgG antitransglutaminase and IgA/IgG antideamidated gliadin peptides, positivity of the latest having a good correlation with gluten exposure.[19] Detection of gluten immunogenic peptides in stool and urine enlarges the possibilities of control GFD.[20,21]

Upper gastrointestinal endoscopy with duodenal biopsies is necessary to confirm RCD and define its type (**Fig. 1**). Double-balloon enteroscopy may be useful, guided by capsule endoscopy in suspicion of RCDII for a better assessment of ulcers, particularly for evidence of ulcerative jejunitis found in roughly 70% of patients.[17,22] Thus, the risk of retention of capsule endoscopy imposes preliminary radiological imaging of the small bowel to rule out strictures. Definitive diagnosis relies on histology. In RCDI, histology is similar to that found in active CD with villus atrophy and increased

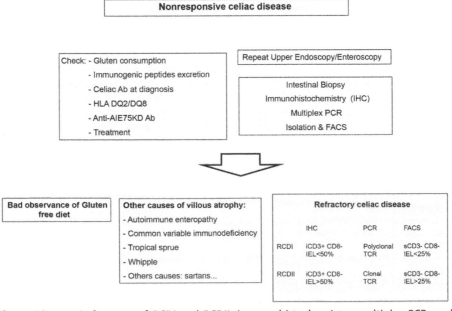

Fig. 1. Diagnostic features of RCDI and RCDII: immunohistochemistry, multiplex PCR, and flow cytometry.

normal intraepithelial lymphocytes (IELs). Molecular analysis showed polyclonal reper- toire. No other diagnostic criteria have been yet defined for RCDI. In contrast, the hall- mark abnormal population, detected by 3 combined techniques, makes the diagnosis of RCDII more specific: more than 25% of the CD103+ or CD45+ IELs lacking surface CD3 T-cell receptor complexes on flow cytometry (**Fig. 2**) or more than 50% of IELs expressing intracellular CD3ε but no CD8 in formalin-fixed sections and/or the pres- ence of a detectable clonal rearrangement of the gamma chain of the T-cell receptor (TCR) in duodenal biopsies (see **Fig. 2**).[23,24] Similar features allow detecting lympho- cytic gastritis and colitis containing the same abnormal population in approximately 50% and 30% of RCDII patients, respectively.[17] NKP46 staining represents a prom- ising diagnostic tool for distinguishing clonal RCDII from RCDI or CD.[25]

Fluorescence-activated cell sorting (FACS) analysis of freshly isolated IELs is partic- ularly useful to distinguish RCDII from other causes of severe enteropathy with villus atrophy and clonal TCRgamma rearrangement, such as granular lymphocytic leukemia, infiltrating intestine of patients with CD[26] or intestinal small CD4 T-cell lym- phoma.[27] Analysis of the delta chain rearrangement may be useful in patients with RCDII presenting oligoclonal rearrangement of the gamma chain.[17] Interest of detect- ing of the beta chain of the TCR has also been suggested.[28,29] Finally, specificity of the polymerase chain reaction (PCR) product needs to be attested by formation of homoduplexes[17] because of prominent clonal peaks possibly found in patients with RCDI or CD.[30]

CLINICAL FEATURES AND OUTCOME

Resistance to a GFD is primary in roughly one-third and one-half patients with RCDI and RCDII, respectively.[17] Symptoms are notably less severe in RCDI than RCDII

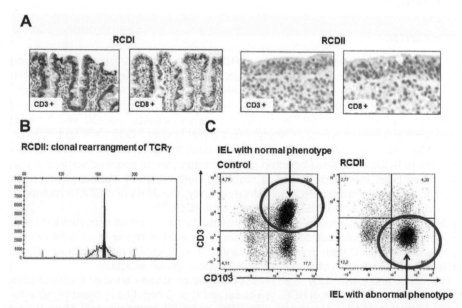

Fig. 2. Investigation of enteropathy with villus atrophy refractory to GFD. (*A*) Immunohisto- chemistry. (*B*) Multiplex PCR. (*C*) Flow cytometry. (*Courtesy of* [A] Virginie Verkarre, MD, Paris, France; and [B] Elizabeth Macintyre, MD, PhD, Paris, France; and [C] Nadine Cerf-Bensussan, MD, PhD, Paris, France; and Nicolas Guegan, PhD, Paris, France.)

frequently associated with protein-losing enteropathy.[17] RCDII is associated with poor prognosis with 5-year survival rates of 44% to 58%.[14,15,17] The more severe malnutrition combined with the higher risk of developing overt lymphoma explains the higher mortality in RCDII than in RCDI.[17] Confirming this hypothesis, decreased albumin and abnormal IEL phenotype are significantly associated with 5-year mortality in a multivariate model to predict survival in refractory CD.[30] Nevertheless, the mortality rate in RCDI appears higher than in uncomplicated CD.[17] One explanation is the lack of curative treatment for RCD. Immunosuppressive drugs have only a poor therapeutic effect and may predispose to overt lymphoma.[31] The second reason is the natural increased risk of developing overt lymphoma (enteropathy-associated T-cell lymphoma [EATL]). Indeed, 33% to 52% of patients with RCDII develop EATL within 5 years after diagnosis.[14,15,17] Onset of EATL in RCDI is not null even if much lower than in RCDII, with a 5-year rate of 14% in the more pessimistic studies.[17] In RCDII, abnormal IELs may be found in mesenteric lymph nodes, blood, bone marrow, and in different epitheliums, such as lung and skin.[17] Extraintestinal dissemination of RCDII IELs explains that EATL does not develop exclusively in the intestine. EATL may notably arise from RCDII cutaneous lesions. Their expression of CD103 and their identical TCRγ clonality[17] ascertain their origin from RCDII IELs. Patients with RCDII require regular clinical follow-up combined with enteroscopy, computed tomography scan or MRI small bowel follow-through and PET scan.[32] PET scan can further guide realization of radiologically guided biopsy or explorative laparoscopy. It must, however, be stressed that EATL can arise in patients with CD who do not display any evidence of RCDII. Histologic diagnosis is easier than in RCDII with infiltration by medium to large lymphoids expressing CD30 in more than 80% of cases.[33] The prognosis of EATL is poor, with an overall survival currently estimated at 20% to 25% 5 years after the diagnosis, with a better diagnosis in EATL complicating CD compared with EATL complicating RCDII.[33,34]

PATHOGENESIS

It remains unknown whether patients with RCD have a particular genetic background differentiating them from patients with uncomplicated CD. It has been reported that severity of celiac disease was correlated with the number of HLA-DQ2 copies: homozygosity for HLA-DQ2 was observed in 25.5% of RCDI, 44.1% of RCD II, and 53.3% of patients with EATL versus 20.7% of uncomplicated patients with CD and 2.1% of controls.[35] In a recent European study, most patients with RCDII were homozygous HLA-DQ2 (>64.4%).[36] Moreover, this study identified the locus 7p14.3 as favoring progression to RCDII.[36] Besides inherited genetic factors, some acquired somatic mutations have been identified. Indeed, a recurrent partial trisomy 1q22-q44 has been found in most patients with RCDII.[37] More recently, the JAK1 and STAT3 mutations were identified in abnormal IELs in patients with RCDII.[38]

Onset of RCD may be favored by environmental factors, such as exposure to gluten. Risk of lymphomatous complications was reported 4 times higher in patients without adherence to a GFD than compliant patients.[3] The scientific rationale may rely on more intense production of interleukin (IL)-15 under gluten exposure.[39]

Infections, and particularly viral infections, may constitute another environmental factor favoring emergence of RCD. We observed B or C hepatitis at onset of refractoriness in 20% and 10% of patients with RCDI or RCDII, respectively.[17] More than a specific virus, it is rather suspected that components of the antiviral responses and, notably, type I interferons might promote the onset of chronic inflammatory disorders (reviewed in Foxman and Iwasaki[40]). Type I interferon may notably stimulate the survival and proliferation of CD8+ T cells and natural killer cells, either directly or via the induction of IL-15.[40] We can hypothesize that such mechanism may occur in RCDI helping the immunologic reaction initiated by gluten to evolve toward autoimmunity. Accordingly, symptoms improve under immunosuppressive treatments.[17] However, mechanisms of RCDI are largely unknown and remain to be substantiated. More progress has been performed recently in the understanding of the pathogenesis of RCDII. Contrary to EATL, which expressed Ki67, RCDII is characterized by massive accumulation of abnormal IEL without in situ detectable proliferation but with apoptosis defect.[39] In active CD and RCDII, IL-15 produced in excess exerts potent antiapoptotic effects that prevent the elimination of activated IELs and promote their massive accumulation by activating a survival signal.[39,40] Indeed, clonal RCDII IELs acquired somatic mutations (JAKI, STAT3) that selectively increase their responsiveness to IL-15. Human anti-IL-15 antibodies inhibit ex vivo the IL-15–driven signaling pathway in intestinal organotypic cultures of patients with RCDII. In vivo, treatment by this antibody of mice overexpressing human IL-15 in small bowel wiped out the IEL hyperplasia observed in these mice.[41]

TREATMENTS

Steroids improved clinical symptoms in most patients with either type of RCD with various histologic response from 30% to 40% of cases to nearly 90% in a recent study using open capsule budesonide.[17,42] Because of steroid dependence, immunosuppressors such as azathioprine or anti-TNF-α are used and produce transient clinical response but rare mucosal improvement.[17] In RCDII, immunosuppressive drugs have no impact on the abnormal clonal IEL population and could enhance the risk of overt lymphoma as observed with azathioprine and anti-CD52 by depletive effect.[17] In RCDI, no scientific rationale has yet been established to treat specifically patients with RCDI with targeted therapy. The nonproliferative RCDII cells are thus difficult to eradicate by regular chemotherapy and may represent a reservoir of cells susceptible to more aggressive transformation. Purine analogues, such as pentostatin or cladribine (2CDA), showed moderate clinical, histologic, and hematological efficacies.[43,44] In our experience, 2CDA can induce clinical and histologic response in patients with RCDII.[17] However, explosive onset of overt lymphoma was observed in the 2 treated patients within 3 to 8 weeks after treatment, precluding further use of these drugs. Another strategy is the use of autologous hematopoietic stem cell transplantation, which induced clinical and histologic response but no sustained reduction of abnormal IELs in the 13 treated patients.[45,46] The use of chemotherapy before autologous hematopoietic stem cell transplantation may probably increase hematological response. Targeted strategy appears necessary to complete the therapeutic armory to treat RCDII. Blocking IL-15 signaling appears the treatment of choice in RCDII.[41] The preliminary results of a phase II clinical trial using the humanized anti-IL-15 antibody are encouraging.[47] Treatment of RCDII will probably combine, in the near future, conventional chemotherapy agents and targeted therapy blocking IL-15 signaling (reviewed in Malamut and colleagues[48]).

SUMMARY

In conclusion, RCD refers to 2 distinct entities: RCDI, the benign form, and the malignant form RCDII characterized by clonal expansion of small aberrant IELs. Small bowel investigations (enteroscopy, videocapsule endoscopy) and specialized techniques of IEL analyses (immunohistochemistry, molecular biology, flow cytometry) are necessary for diagnosis of both forms of RCD. Prognosis of RCDII is severe due to malnutrition and high risk of overt lymphoma. Recent advances in understanding the pathogenesis of refractory celiac disease open the possibility of targeted therapy.

ACKNOWLEDGMENTS

The authors thank Nadine Cerf-Bensussan (Inserm UMR1163, Institut Imagine) for FACS analysis of normal and abnormal IELs, Nicole Brousse (Anatomopathology Necker, Université Paris Descartes) for immunohistochemistry, and Elisabeth Macintyre (Biological Hematology, Hôpital Necker Enfants Malades, Paris) for providing example of Multiplex PCR. The authors acknowledge the INCa (Institut National du Cancer) Netwok CELAC (Centre Expert National des Lymphomes Associés à la maladie Coeliaque).

REFERENCES

1. Thomason K, West J, Logan RF, et al. Fracture experience of patients with coeliac disease: a population based survey. Gut 2003;52:518–22.
2. Cosnes J, Cellier C, Viola S, et al. Incidence of autoimmune diseases in celiac disease: protective effect of the gluten-free diet. Clin Gastroenterol Hepatol 2008;6:753–8.
3. Holmes GK, Prior P, Lane MR, et al. Malignancy in coeliac disease–effect of a gluten free diet. Gut 1989;30:333–8.
4. Lebwohl B, Murray JA, Rubio-Tapia A, et al. Predictors of persistent villus atrophy in coeliac disease: a population-based study. Aliment Pharmacol Ther 2014;39: 488–95.
5. Lebwohl B, Michaelsson K, Green PH, et al. Persistent mucosal damage and risk of fracture in celiac disease. J Clin Endocrinol Metab 2014;99:609–16.
6. Lebwohl B, Granath F, Ekbom A, et al. Mucosal healing and risk for lymphoproliferative malignancy in celiac disease: a population-based cohort study. Ann Intern Med 2013;159:169–75.
7. Vahedi K, Mascart F, Mary JY, et al. Reliability of antitransglutaminase antibodies as predictors of gluten-free diet compliance in adult celiac disease. Am J Gastroenterol 2003;98:1079–87.
8. Akram S, Murray JA, Pardi DS, et al. Adult autoimmune enteropathy: Mayo Clinic Rochester experience. Clin Gastroenterol Hepatol 2007;5:1282–90.
9. Khokhar N, Gill ML. Tropical sprue: revisited. J Pak Med Assoc 2004;54:133–4.
10. Malamut G, Verkarre V, Suarez F, et al. The enteropathy associated with common variable immunodeficiency: the delineated frontiers with celiac disease. Am J Gastroenterol 2010;105:2262–75.
11. Scialom S, Malamut G, Meresse B, et al. Gastrointestinal disorder associated with olmesartan mimics autoimmune enteropathy. PLoS One 2015;10(6):e0125024.
12. Roshan B, Leffler DA, Jamma S, et al. The incidence and clinical spectrum of refractory celiac disease in a North American referral center. Am J Gastroenterol 2011;106:923–8.
13. West J. Celiac disease and its complications: a time traveller's perspective. Gastroenterology 2009;136:32–4.
14. Rubio-Tapia A, Kelly DG, Lahr BD, et al. Clinical staging and survival in refractory celiac disease: a single center experience. Gastroenterology 2009;136:99–107.
15. Al-Toma A, Verbeek WH, Hadithi M, et al. Survival in refractory coeliac disease and enteropathy associated T cell lymphoma: retrospective evaluation of single centre experience. Gut 2007;56:1373–8.

16. Daum S, Cellier C, Mulder CJ. Refractory coeliac disease. Best Pract Res Clin Gastroenterol 2005;19:413–24.
17. Malamut G, Afchain P, Verkarre V, et al. Presentation and long-term follow-up of refractory celiac disease: comparison of type I with type II. Gastroenterology 2009;136:81–90.
18. Malamut G, Cellier C. Is refractory celiac disease more severe in old Europe? Am J Gastroenterol 2011;106:929–32.
19. de Chaisemartin L, Meatchi T, Malamut G, et al. Application of deamidated gliadin antibodies in the follow-up of treated celiac disease. PLoS One 2015; 10(8):e0136745.
20. Comino I, Fernández-Bañares F, Esteve M, et al. Fecal gluten peptides reveal limitations of serological tests and food questionnaires for monitoring gluten-free diet in celiac disease patients. Am J Gastroenterol 2016;111(10):1456–65.
21. Moreno ML, Cebolla Á, Muñoz-Suano A, et al. Detection of gluten immunogenic peptides in the urine of patients with coeliac disease reveals transgressions in the gluten-free diet and incomplete mucosal healing. Gut 2017;66:250–7.
22. Barret MMG, Rahmi G, Samaha A, et al. Diagnostic yield of capsule endoscopy in refractory celiac disease. Am J Gastroenterol 2012;107(10):1546–53.
23. Cellier C, Patey N, Mauvieux L, et al. Abnormal intestinal intraepithelial lymphocytes In refractory sprue. Gastroenterology 1998;114:471–81.
24. Cellier C, Delabesse E, Helmer C, et al. Refractory sprue, coeliac disease, and enteropathy-associated T-cell lymphoma. French Coeliac Disease Study Group. Lancet 2000;356:203–8.
25. Cheminant M, Bruneau J, Malamut G, et al. NKP46 is a useful diagnostic biomarker in gastrointestinal T-cell lymphoproliferative diseases. A CELAC network study. ICDS (17th International Celiac disease symposium) New Delhi, India, September 2017.
26. Malamut G, Meresse B, Verkarre V, et al. Large Granular Lymphocytic Leukemia complicating Celiac disease: a rare cause of refractory celiac disease. Gastroenterology 2012;143:1470–2.
27. Malamut G, Meresse B, Kaltenbach S, et al. Small intestinal CD4+ T-cell lymphoma is a heterogenous entity with common pathology features. Clin Gastroenterol Hepatol 2014;12(4):599–608.
28. Perfetti V, Brunetti L, Biagi F, et al. TCRbeta clonality improves diagnostic yield of TCRgamma clonality in refractory celiac disease. J Clin Gastroenterol 2012;46: 675–9.
29. Ritter J, Zimmermann K, Jöhrens K, et al. T-cell repertoires in refractory coeliac disease. Gut 2018;67(4):644–53.
30. Hussein S, Gindin T, Lagana SM, et al. Clonal T cell receptor gene rearrangements in coeliac disease: implications for diagnosing refractory coeliac disease. J Clin Pathol 2018;71(9):825–31.
31. Goerres MS, Meijer JW, Wahab PJ, et al. Azathioprine and prednisone combination therapy in refractory coeliac disease. Aliment Pharmacol Ther 2003;18: 487–94.
32. Hoffmann M, Vogelsang H, Kletter K, et al. 18F-fluoro-deoxy-glucose positron emission tomography (18F-FDG-PET) for assessment of enteropathy-type T cell lymphoma. Gut 2003;52:347–51.
33. Malamut G, Chandesris O, Verkarre V, et al. Enteropathy associated T cell lymphoma in celiac disease: a large retrospective study. Dig Liver Dis 2013;45: 377–84.

34. Gale J, Simmonds PD, Mead GM, et al. Enteropathy-type intestinal T-cell lymphoma: clinical features and treatment of 31 patients in a single center. J Clin Oncol 2000;18:795–803.
35. Al-Toma A, Goerres MS, Meijer JW, et al. Human leukocyte antigen-DQ2 homozygosity and the development of refractory celiac disease and enteropathy-associated T-cell lymphoma. Clin Gastroenterol Hepatol 2006;4:315–9.
36. Hrdlickova B, Mulder C, Malamut G, et al. A locus at 7p14.3 predisposes to refractory celiac disease progression from celiac disease. Eur J Gastroenterol Hepatol 2018;30(8):828–37.
37. Verkarre V, Romana SP, Cellier C, et al. Recurrent partial trisomy 1q22-q44 in clonal intraepithelial lymphocytes in refractory celiac sprue. Gastroenterology 2003;125:40–6.
38. Ettersperger J, Montcuquet N, Malamut G, et al. Interleukin-15-dependent T-cell-like innate intraepithelial lymphocytes develop in the intestine and transform into lymphomas in celiac disease. Immunity 2016;45(3):610–25.
39. Mention JJ, Ben Ahmed M, Begue B, et al. Interleukin 15: a key to disrupted intraepithelial lymphocyte homeostasis and lymphomagenesis in celiac disease. Gastroenterology 2003;125:730–45.
40. Foxman EF, Iwasaki A. Genome-virome interactions: examining the role of common viral infections in complex disease. Nat Rev Microbiol 2011;4:254–64.
41. Malamut G, El Machhour R, Montcuquet N, et al. IL-15 triggers an antiapoptotic pathway in human intraepithelial lymphocytes that is a potential new target in celiac disease-associated inflammation and lymphomagenesis. J Clin Invest 2010; 120:2131–43.
42. Mukewar SS, Sharma A, Rubio-Tapia A, et al. Open-capsule budesonide for refractory celiac disease. Am J Gastroenterol 2017;112(6):959–67.
43. Dray X, Joly F, Lavergne-Slove A, et al. A severe but reversible refractory sprue. Gut 2006;55:1210–1.
44. Al-Toma A, Goerres MS, Meijer JW, et al. Cladribine therapy in refractory celiac disease with aberrant T cells. Clin Gastroenterol Hepatol 2006;4:1322–7.
45. Al-Toma A, Visser OJ, van Roessel HM, et al. Autologous hematopoietic stem cell transplantation in refractory celiac disease with aberrant T-cells. Blood 2007; 109(5):2243–9.
46. Tack GJ, Wondergem MJ, Al-Toma A, et al. Auto-SCT in refractory celiac disease type II patients unresponsive to cladribine therapy. Bone Marrow Transplant 2011;46(6):840–6.
47. Cellier C, Bouma G, van Gils T, et al. AMG 714 (anti-IL-15 Mab) halts the progression of aberrant intraepithelial lymphocytes in refractory celiac disease type II (RCDII): a phase 2A randomized, double blind, placebo-controlled study evaluating AMG714 in adult patients with RCDII/pre-EATL. Washington, DC: DDW; 2018.
48. Malamut G, Meresse B, Cellier C, et al. Refractory celiac disease: from bench to bedside. Semin Immunopathol 2012;34(4):601–13.

Nondietary Therapies for Celiac Disease

Gloria Serena, PhD[a,b], Ciaran P. Kelly, MD[b,c], Alessio Fasano, MD[a,b],*

KEYWORDS

- Gluten • Endopeptidases • Immune response • Intestinal permeability

KEY POINTS

- A strictly gluten-free diet (GFD) is effective in treating celiac disease.
- The GFD is challenging and difficult to maintain.
- Nondietary therapies are needed to reduce the burden of treatment in celiac disease, especially for patients with nonresponsive or refractory celiac disease, for which the GFD alone is not effective.
- Many of the sequential steps in celiac disease pathogenesis are well elucidated, hence there are multiple well-defined targets for research and drug development.
- Attractive treatment options include enzymatic gluten degradation, binding and sequestration of gluten, restoration of epithelial tight junction barrier function, inhibition of tissue transglutaminase 2 or of human leukocyte antigen–mediated gliadin peptide presentation, and induction of tolerance to gluten.

INTRODUCTION

Celiac disease (CD) is an autoimmune enteropathy triggered by gluten in genetically predisposed individuals carrying human leukocyte antigen (HLA) DQ2 and/or DQ8.[1] At present, the gold standard treatment of CD is a lifelong gluten-free diet (GFD). However, a small percentage of patients have refractory CD and do not respond

Disclosure: A. Fasano is a stock holder of Alba Therapeutics, a company producing celiac disease treatments alternative to the gluten-free diet. C.P. Kelly has received grant funding from Allergan; is a scientific advisor for Immunogenx, Innovate, and Takeda Pharmaceuticals; and is a scientific advisor for and stock holder of Cour Pharma and Glutenostics. G. Serena has nothing to disclose.
[a] Division of Pediatric Gastroenterology and Nutrition, Mucosal Immunology and Biology Research Center, MassGeneral Hospital for Children, 175 Cambridge Street, CPZS – 574, Boston, MA 02114, USA; [b] Celiac Research Program, Harvard Medical School, 25 Shattuck Street, Boston, MA 02115, USA; [c] Department of Medicine, Division of Gastroenterology, Beth Israel Deaconess Medical Center, 330 Brookline Avenue, Boston, MA 02215, USA
* Corresponding author. Celiac Research Program, Harvard Medical School, Mucosal Immunology and Biology Research Center, MassGeneral Hospital for Children, 175 Cambridge Street, CPZS – 574, Boston, MA 02114.
E-mail address: AFASANO@mgh.harvard.edu

Gastroenterol Clin N Am 48 (2019) 145–163
https://doi.org/10.1016/j.gtc.2018.09.011
0889-8553/19/© 2018 Elsevier Inc. All rights reserved.

to dietary treatment.[2] Given the limited nutritional value of gluten, its elimination from the diet is considered safe. However, the consumption of some nutrients may be reduced in patients on a GFD.[1] Furthermore, following a strict GFD can still be psychologically and socially challenging because of its restrictive nature.[3] These challenges are compounded by the cost of gluten-free food and the persistent risk of hidden gluten while traveling or eating in public spaces.[4–8] For these reasons, the demand for nondietary alternative treatments for CD is increasing among patients and clinicians. Novel potential nondietary therapies have been proposed and are being evaluated in clinical trials thanks to progress made during the past few years concerning CD pathogenesis.

Innate immune cells have been reported to play a role in the first stages of the disease. Interleukin (IL)-15 production is increased in patients with untreated CD upon ingestion of gluten[9] (**Fig. 1**). It triggers the polarization of dendritic cells (DCs) or monocytes toward a proinflammatory phenotype[9] and alters the function of T cell receptor

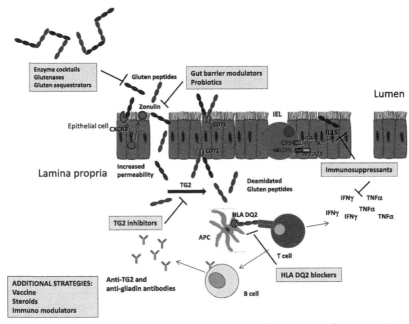

Fig. 1. Proposed interventional approaches targeting the factors contributing to CD pathogenesis. Gluten fragments are resistant to gastrointestinal breakdown by luminal and brush border enzymes. Use of enzyme cocktails, glutenases, and gluten inhibitors could reduce the exposure to immunogenic gluten peptides. At the intestinal epithelium level, increased intestinal permeability enables the paracellular and transcellular translocation of gluten peptides into the lamina propria. Probiotics and gut barrier modulators reduce the alteration in intestinal permeability. Gluten peptides induce production of IL-15, resulting in an increase in the number of intraepithelial lymphocytes (IELs) and apoptosis and triggering the activation of MICA/B-NKG2D and CD94/NKG2C-HLA-E. Neutralizing IL-15–mediated effects could reduce the inflammation in patients with CD. Gluten peptides are deamidated by transglutaminase 2 (TG2) and then recognized by CD4+ T cells in the context of HLA-DQ2/DQ8. Thus, either TG2 inhibitors or HLA blockers are proposed as potential drug candidates. Immunosuppressants could suppress the T-cell and B-cell response in the mucosa. Additional means to prevent or treat CD are vaccines, immunomodulators, or steroids. APC, antigen-presenting cell; IFN, interferon; TNF, tumor necrosis factor.

alpha beta (TCRαβ) intraepithelial lymphocytes (IELs) in the epithelium, resulting in the destruction of the intestinal tissue.[10] Similarly, interferon (IFN) alfa expression is dysregulated in patients with CD and promotes natural killer (NK) cell, CD8+ T cell, and DC activation.[11] Neutrophil infiltration characterizes the initial dysregulated immune response to gluten,[12] and IL-8 has been shown to be released by the epithelium and immune cells of patients with CD on stimulation with gluten.[13,14] In vitro studies have shown that gliadin triggers production of tumor necrosis factor α (TNF-α), IL-8, RANTES, IL-1β, and nitric oxide from macrophages.[9,15] In addition, alpha-amylase trypsin inhibitors have been reported to activate innate immune cells by engaging toll-like receptor 2 (TLR2), myeloid differentiation factor 2 (MD2), and CD14 (cluster of differentiation 14) complex.[15] The role of innate lymphoid cells in the pathogenesis of CD has not been completely elucidated yet; however, their increased number in the mucosa of patients with CD suggests their involvement in the initiation of tolerance loss as well.[16]

The adaptive immune response in CD is initiated by antigen-presenting cells carrying gluten peptides to CD4+ T cells, leading to their activation and triggering the release of proinflammatory cytokines and the production of metalloproteases and keratinocyte growth factor by stromal cells.[17] T-helper (Th) 1 cells represent the major mediators of the mucosal immune response to gliadin.[18] The presence of Th17 cytokines has suggested the contribution of Th17-mediated inflammatory response in the pathogenesis of CD as well.[19] In addition, the high expression of IL-15 on enterocytes in active CD has been shown contribute to the overexpression of the NK receptors CD94 and NK group 2 member D (NKG2D) by CD3+ IELs[18] (see **Fig. 1**).

Alterations in the T-regulatory cell (T_{reg}) populations are associated with the onset of CD as well. T_{regs} have been shown to be more numerous in active patients with CD and present an impaired suppressive function compared with cells from healthy controls.[20] Furthermore, a recent study has reported a link between the Th17-mediated immune response and epigenetic defects on T_{regs} from patients with CD.[21]

Along with defects in the immune machinery, alterations in the intestinal stem cell compartment have been suggested to contribute to the cascade of events that leads to CD. A recent study has shown expansion of the immature progenitor cell compartment and downregulation of the Hedgehog signaling pathway that may contribute to the hyperplasic crypt that characterizes CD.[22]

Given the remarkable increase of CD prevalence worldwide, it has been suggested that environmental factors may contribute to the loss of tolerance in genetically predisposed individuals.[23–29] Alterations in the intestinal microbiome have been described in numerous studies and evidence for the role of dysbiosis in the onset of CD is growing. Although the exact contribution of the microbiome in the development of CD has not been fully elucidated, in vitro studies have shown that proinflammatory cytokines abundantly produced in patients with CD trigger changes in the microbial composition.[30]

Potential Alternative/Adjuvant Treatment to the Gluten-Free Diet

Having a more in-depth understanding of the steps leading to the break of tolerance to gluten and the onset of CD provided several possible targets for treatments alternative/complementary to the GFD (see **Fig. 1**). Since 2005, when the first trial was registered on clinicaltrials.gov, there have been 192 registered trials, of which 43 focused on specific treatment alternatives to the GFD (**Fig. 2**). These treatments, focused on 6 specific technologies, are integrated by another 5 technologies that are either in the preclinical phase of development or have been developed for other indications and are now applied to CD (**Table 1**).

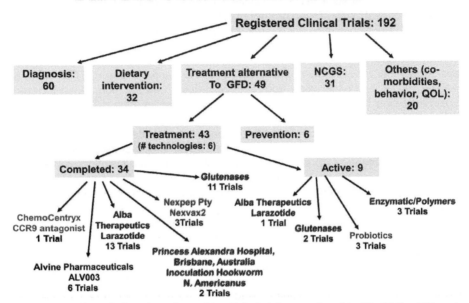

Fig. 2. Overall list of all trials registered in clinicaltrials.gov related to CD. Of the 192 registered clinical trials, 49 are related to treatments alternative/integrative to the GFD (43 trials related to 6 technologies) or disease prevention (6 trials). CCR9, C-C chemokine receptor 9; NCGS, nonceliac gluten sensitivity; QOL, quality of life.

Enzyme cocktails

A major peculiarity of gliadins and glutenins is their high content of proline and glutamine amino acid residues, which make human digestive enzymes (both intraluminal and brush border proteases) ineffective in completely digesting these proteins. This incomplete digestion leaves large proline-rich gluten fragments intact, including immunogenic (33-mer from α-gliadin and a 26-mer from γ-gliadin) epitopes. These latter peptides can trigger proinflammatory T-cell responses resulting in the tissue remodeling typical of CD enteropathy. Proline endopeptidases have been shown to effectively degrade the immunogenic gluten peptides in vitro and, therefore, have been proposed as oral supplements. Several existing digestive enzyme supplements also claim to aid in gluten degradation and have been commercialized with this claim. However, they have never been rigorously tested to establish their efficacy. A recent study compared 5 commercially available digestive enzyme supplements along with purified digestive enzymes in their effectiveness in degrading toxic gluten epitopes monitored by R5 enzyme-linked immunosorbent assay (ELISA), mass spectrometric analysis of the degradation products, and T-cell proliferation assays.[31] The digestive enzyme supplements showed comparable proteolytic activities and very limited gluten detoxification properties as determined by ELISA. Mass spectrometric analysis of these products showed the presence of many different amylases and a variety of different proteases with aminopeptidase and carboxypeptidase activity. However, the enzyme supplements left the 9 immunogenic epitopes of the 26-mer and 33-mer gliadin fragments largely intact. T-cell proliferation assays confirmed the mass spectrometric data, showing unaffected T-cell activation following treatment

Table 1

Classes of compounds and molecules proposed for prevention and/or treatment of Celiac disease used in ongoing or completed clinical trials

Class	Mechanism of Action	Compound	Company	Status	Number of Subjects Tested	Number of Articles Published
Glutenases	Glutenase	ALV003	Alvine, United States	Phase IIb	829	2
	Glutenase	AN-PEP	DSM, Netherlands	Phase I + II	14	1
	Glutenase	STAN1	Heim Pal Children's Hospital, Hungary	Phase I + II	38	0
Enzymes cocktail	Pancrelipase	Creon	Sheffield Teaching Hospitals, United Kingdom	Phase IV	2	0
Gluten sequestrators	Gluten-sequestering polymers	P(HEMA-co-SS) (BL-7010)	University of Montreal, Canada	Phase I + II	40	0
Probiotics	Gluten tolerization	*Bifidobacterium infantis*	University of Buenos Aires, Argentina	Exploratory	42	0
	Gluten tolerization	Genetically modified *Lactococcus lactis*	ActoGenix, Belgium	Discovery	NA	—
Gut barrier stabilizer	Zonulin antagonist	AT-1001	Alba, United States	Phase IIb	785	5
tTG2 inhibitors	TG2 inhibitor	Dihydroisoxazoles	Sitari Pharmaceuticals	Discovery	NA	1
	TG2 inhibitor	ZED-101	Zedira, Germany	Discovery	NA	0
	TG2 inhibitor	Cinnamoyl triazoles	University of Montreal, Canada	Discovery	NA	1
HLA-DQ2 blockers	HLA-DQ2 blocker	Dimeric analogue of gluten peptide	Stanford University, United States and University of Oslo, Norway	Discovery	NA	1
	HLA-DQ2 blocker	Azidoproline analogue of gluten peptide	Leiden University, Netherlands	Discovery	NA	1
Immune modulators	CCR9 antagonist	CCX282-B	ChemoCentryx, United States	Phase II	90	0
	Immune modulation	*Necator americanus*	Princess Alexandra Hospital, Australia	Phase II	92	2

(continued on next page)

Table 1
(continued)

Class	Mechanism of Action	Compound	Company	Status	Number of Subjects Tested	Number of Articles Published
Steroids	Topical steroid	Budesonide	Generic drug	Approved	NA	7
	Topical steroid	Prednisolone	Generic drug	Phase II–III	33	7
Immune suppressants	Anti-IL-15	AMG 714	Amgen, United States	Phase II in RA (discon.)	92	0
	Anti-IFN-γ	Fontolizumab	PDL and Biogen Idec, United States	Phase II in IBD (discon.)	NA	0
	Anti-CD3	Visilizumab	Facet, United States	Phase II in UC, GvHD (discon.)	NA	0
	Anti-CD3	Teplizumab	MacroGenes, United States	Phase II in T1D	NA	0
	Anti-CD3	Otelixizumab	Tolerx, United States	Approved	NA	0
	Anti-CD20	Rituximab	Biogen Idec, United States	Approved	NA	0
	Anti-CD20	Tositumomab	GlaxoSmithKline, United States	Approved	NA	0
	Anti-CD20	Ibritumomab	Spectrum, United States	Approved	NA	0
	Anti–TNF-α	Infliximab	Janssen Biotech, United States	Approved	121	0
	Anti–TNF-α	Certolizumab	UCB, United States	Approved	NA	0
	Anti–TNF-α	Adalimumab	AbbVie, United States	Approved	NA	0
	Anti-integrinα4β7	Vedolizumab	Millennium Pharmaceuticals, United States	Phase II	10	9
	IL-2/IL-15R beta	Hu-Mik-Beta1	National Cancer Institute, United States	Phase I	12	3
	Antigluten	AGY	IgY, Canada	Phase I	10	0
Vaccine	Peptide vaccination	Nexvax2	NexPep, Australia	Phase I	86	1

Abbreviations: CCR9, C-C chemokine receptor 9; GvHD, graft-versus-host disease; IBD, inflammatory bowel disease; NA, not available; P(HEMA-co-SS), poly(hydroxyethylmethacrylate-co-styrene sulfonate); tTG2, tissue transglutaminase 2; UC, ulcerative colitis.

Data from National Institute of Health: US National Library of Medicine. Clinicaltrials.gov. Available at: https://clinicaltrials.gov/. Accessed June 7, 2018.

with these supplements. These results refute the unproven claims for these products in detoxifying gluten and confirm the major risk in using products that have not undergone rigorous clinical testing to prove safety and efficacy of any given remedy intended for treatment, amelioration, or prevention of diseases such as CD.

These concerns are confirmed by a study from Krishnareddy and colleagues[32] that investigated the contents, claims, and disclaimers of commercially available glutenase products and assessed patient interest using Google AdWords to obtain Google search frequencies. The investigators evaluated 14 glutenase products, all containing proteases, including X-prolyl exopeptidase dipeptidyl peptidase IV (8 products), whereas the remaining products either did not state the protease contents (2), or failed to specify the name or origin of all proteases (8). Eleven contained carbohydrases and lipases and 3 contained probiotics. Thirteen out of 14 claimed to degrade immunogenic gluten fragments, and 4 claimed to help alleviate gastrointestinal symptoms associated with eating gluten. Disclaimers included not being evaluated by the US Food and Drug Administration and products not intended to diagnose, treat, cure, or prevent any disease. On Google AdWords, the search frequency for the product names and the search terms was 3173 searches per month. This study provides another example of how the commercial names of these products make implicit claims on the labels and Web sites, but these are not supported by any scientific basis. What is even more concerning is that Google search data suggest great interest and therefore possible use by patients with CD who perceive these products as proven remedies for ameliorating the consequences of inadvertent or purposeful gluten ingestion.

Propyl endopeptidases (glutenases)
Gluten proteins from wheat, barley, and rye capable of activating CD-associated T-cell responses have high prolamine and glutamine contents and are resistant to degradation by human digestive endopeptidases and exopeptidases. They are also highly resistant to cooking, even at high temperatures. Partial proteolysis of gluten proteins generates oligopeptide fragments, such as the 33-mer and 26-mer peptides discussed earlier, that are modified by tissue transglutaminase (TTG), bind HLA DQ2/8, and potently activate gliadin-specific T cells. To interrupt this sequence and degrade gliadin to smaller, nonimmunogenic fragments, propyl endopeptidases (PEPs) from plants and microorganisms have been used to supplement the inadequate repertoire of human digestive enzymes. PEP digestion can be achieved by predigestion of dietary gluten before consumption or by digestion in the stomach and proximal small intestine after ingestion. The latter is more attractive as a therapeutic/preventive application, but substantial challenges exist in terms of PEP stability and enzymatic activity in the wide pH ranges of the stomach and duodenum as well as the ability to promptly access and degrade gluten that is embedded in a complex food matrix.

Latiglutenase Latiglutenase (formerly ALV003) is the glutenase pair that has been most extensively studied in human clinical trials to date. Latiglutenase consists of a 1:1 ratio of ALV001, a modified recombinant cysteine endoprotease from barley (EP-B2), and ALV002, a modified recombinant bacterial PEP from S capsulate (SC-PEP).[33]

ALV003 has completed several phase I and phase II human trials. In a phase I study, ALV003 predigestion of a gluten-containing meal led to a subsequent reduction in peripheral blood T-cell IFN-γ ELISpot (enzyme-linked immunospot) responses to gliadin.[34] However, symptoms caused by the gluten challenge meal were not alleviated. Two phase I studies found that orally administered latiglutenase is well tolerated and no substantial safety concerns have emerged.[34] Gastric aspirates collected 30 min following the ingestion of 1 g of wheat bread gluten showed that oral latiglutenase 100 and 300 mg degraded 75% and 88% of the gluten respectively. A subsequent phase II study investigated the ability of oral latiglutenase to protect patients with treated CD from mucosal injury caused by gluten challenge (2 g/d for 6 weeks).[35] Duodenal biopsies taken after the gluten challenge showed mucosal injury (including reduced villus height to crypt depth ratio) in the placebo group but no significant mucosal damage in the latiglutenase group.

A subsequent, larger (n = 494) phase II study examined the effects of oral latiglutenase on mucosal morphometric abnormalities in biopsies from patients with nonresponsive CD despite following a GFD for at least 1 year.[36] Patients were assigned randomly to receive placebo or latiglutenase (100–900 mg/d for 12 or 24 weeks). The primary end point was a change in the villus height/crypt depth ratio but there were no significant differences between latiglutenase and placebo groups in this outcome measure. All groups, including placebo, had significant improvements both in histologic and in symptom scores, indicating a trial effect of more stringent dietary gluten avoidance. A post hoc subgroup analysis of the data from this study found a reduction in celiac-related symptoms in TTG-seropositive subjects that was most evident in those receiving the highest dose of latiglutenase (900 mg).[37] This finding opens the way for additional evaluation of latiglutenase in selected patients at highest risk for continued gluten exposure (as shown by positive TTG serology).

Other glutenases A PEP from *Flavobacterium meningosepticum* was used to pretreat gluten as part of a randomized, double-blind study in patients with treated CD.[38] Gluten challenge (5 g/d for 14 days) was performed using either untreated gluten or gluten pretreated with the PEP using a crossover study design. Symptoms were similar regardless of the type of gluten consumed. However, malabsorption of fat, determined by 72-hour quantitative fecal fat, and xylose, determined by D-xylose excretion in urine, was less common during challenge with the PEP-treated gluten.

A bacterial PEP, derived from *Aspergillus niger* (AN-PEP), was shown to remain stable at pH 2 with optimal enzymatic activity at pH 4 to 5 and to effectively digest gluten to nonimmunogenic fragments in an in vitro system designed to model the human gastrointestinal tract.[39,40]

Using molecular modeling, an acid-active endopeptidase from the acidophilic bacterium *Alicyclobacillus sendaiensis* was redesigned to optimize its ability to degrade gluten in the human upper gastrointestinal tract.[41] The resulting protease (Kuma030), recognizes tripeptide sequences in the immunogenic regions of the prolamines of wheat (gliadins), rye (secalins) and barley (hordeins). Kuma030 was reported to degrade greater than 99% of the immunogenic gliadin fraction in vitro in conditions similar to those of the human stomach.[42] Gliadin degradation by Kuma030 effectively eliminated gliadin-dependent T-cell activation. This engineered endopeptidase is now entering human clinical trials as a potential oral therapy for CD.

Gluten sequestrators

Polymer binders have been proposed for the sequestration of gluten in the digestive tract, so preventing its interaction with the gut mucosal and, consequently, all the downstream events leading to immune system engagement and CD activation. One of these polymers, P(HEMA-co-SS) [poly(hydroxyethylmethacrylate-co-styrene sulfonate)] has been shown to reduce the formation of toxic peptides associated with CD by sequestering gluten and so preventing its degradation to toxic, immunogenic peptides.[43] In gluten-sensitized mice, P(HEMA-co-SS) reduced paracellular permeability, normalized the content of antigliadin immunoglobulin A in intestinal washes, and modulated the systemic immune response to gluten in a food mixture. In addition, incubation of P(HEMA-co-SS) with mucosal biopsy specimens from patients with CD decreased the secretion of TNF-α in the presence of partially digested gliadin. In addition, when tested in vivo in a murine model, the copolymer was safe, active regardless of the pH of the environment, and the systemic exposition following oral administration was minimal. These preclinical studies indicate that gluten sequestrators are a possible strategy to ameliorate the risk of dietary gluten cross-contamination; however, their efficacy remains to be tested in clinical trials.

A similar proposed mechanism of action applies to the production and oral administration of antigliadin immunoglobulins designed to bind to gluten contaminating foodstuffs. Bovine colostral immunoglobulin (Ig) G from cows previously immunized against gliadin have been produced and subjected to preclinical testing.[44] Similarly, studies have demonstrated that IgY antibody purified from egg yolks of chickens immunized with gluten can prevent inflammatory and permeability changes induced by gliadin in cultured Caco-2 intestinal epithelial cells and also reduce gliadin absorption in mice.[45,46] A phase I trial has been conducted to assess the safety and efficacy of 1 g of antigliadin IgY with each meal in patients with nonresponsive CD (NCT01765647); publication of results is awaited.

Probiotics bacteria and nematodes

The use of probiotics as a source of endopeptidases to detoxify nondigestible gluten epitopes has been explored by several groups. Certain selected lactobacilli added to sourdough for fermentation have been shown to lyse the proline/glutamine-rich gluten peptides, reducing their immunotoxicity.[47] Fermentation of wheat flour with sourdough lactobacilli or with selected lactobacilli and fungal proteases (routinely used in bakeries) led to a decrease in the concentration of gluten to less than 10 ppm (gluten free).[48] The efficacy of this approach has been tested in vivo by challenging patients with CD in remission with 200 g/d of probiotic-predigested sweet baked goods equivalent to 10 g of native gluten. None of the patients showed worsening in hematological, serologic parameters, or intestinal permeability during 60 days of challenge. This study showed that a wheat flour–fermented product, having gluten completely degraded, is not toxic for patients with CD.[49] In another study, patients with CD were randomly assigned to consumption of 200 g/d of natural flour baked goods (NFBG) (80–127 ppm gluten), extensively hydrolyzed flour baked goods (S1BG) (2480 ppm residual gluten), or fully hydrolyzed baked goods (S2BG) (8 ppm residual gluten) for 60 days.[50] All patients in the NFBG group had symptoms, increased levels of anti-TTG antibodies, and onset of CD enteropathy. The patients who ate the S1BG goods had no clinical complaints but developed subtotal villus atrophy. The patients who were exposed to S2BG had no clinical complaints; their levels of anti-tTG antibodies did not increase, and their Marsh grades of small intestinal mucosa did not change.[50]

Among probiotic preparations, VSL#3, a mixture of 8 lactic acid bacteria and bifidobacteria, has been shown to hydrolyze completely the α2-gliadin–derived epitopes 62–75 and 33-mer peptide and also exerted the capability to increase the epithelial barrier function by stabilizing tight junctions.[51,52]

Complementary to the endopeptidases activities, probiotics have been also considered as a tool to ameliorate gluten-induced inflammation by affecting the host immune function. As mentioned earlier, there is now growing evidence that changes in gut microbiota composition and function may play a key role in CD pathogenesis by epigenetically influencing the host immune system and, therefore, the immune response following gluten exposure. This observation justifies the rationale to explore the use of probiotics to rectify/ameliorate the impact of dysbiosis in CD clinical outcome. To this goal of inducing gluten tolerance, both conventional probiotics (*Bifidobacterium infantis*) and genetically modified probiotics (*Lactococcus lactis*) have been tested in preclinical studies showing some promising initial results (see **Table 1**).

Another interesting approach modulating the immunologic response triggered by gluten exposure is the exposure of patients with CD to parasites in order to facilitate the Th2-dependent immunologic reaction, at the same time inhibiting the Th1-dependent reaction induced by gluten. A double-blind, placebo-controlled, 21-day study conducted by Daveson and colleagues[53] involved patients with CD in remission who were intradermally vaccinated twice with larvae of a hookworm (*Necator americanus*). In week 20 they were orally administered 16 g of gluten daily for 5 days. No differences were observed in the inflammatory parameters and the clinical and histologic picture between the infected and noninfected subjects. The samples drawn from the infected patients showed decreased production of proinflammatory cytokines (IL-17A, INF-γ). However, no effect of infection was observed on the response of the anti–gliadin peptide lymphocytes. Based on these results, this approach seems to be questionable and does not support further investigation on hookworm infection in patients with CD.

Gut barrier stabilizer

Active CD is associated with increased intestinal permeability and reduced tight junction barrier function. These properties expose the subepithelial compartment to proinflammatory luminal contents including microbial products and immunodominant gluten peptides that activate innate and adaptive immune responses. Zonulin, a prehaptoglobin-2 precursor, is believed to modulate epithelial tight junctions and intestinal permeability and is overexpressed in the intestine in active CD.[54–56]

Larazotide acetate Larazotide acetate (formerly AT-1001) is a synthetic octapeptide with a sequence analogous to a portion of *Vibrio cholerae* zonula occludens toxin. In cultured intestinal epithelial monolayers, larazotide acetate enhanced tight junction assembly and barrier function, reduced permeability responses to gliadin fragments and to proinflammatory cytokines, and prevented gluten translocation across the epithelium.[57,58] Larazotide acetate also inhibited gliadin-induced macrophage accumulation and preserved tight junction structure in vivo in gliadin-sensitized HLA-HCD4/DQ8 double transgenic mice.[58]

A small, double-blind, randomized, placebo-controlled pilot study of larazotide acetate used a single 12-mg dose in patients with CD receiving a gluten challenge. Intestinal permeability was measured by fractional urinary excretions of lactulose (LA) and mannitol (MA).[59] Larazotide acetate was well tolerated and seemed to be safe, and its excellent safety history has persisted through all of the additional clinical studies outlined later. Subjects receiving larazotide acetate showed less intestinal permeability dysfunction and IFN-γ production, and fewer gastrointestinal symptoms in response to gluten challenge compared with placebo control subjects.

Three phase II studies of larazotide acetate have been completed and published; the first 2 of these evaluated larazotide acetate in patients with CD undergoing gluten challenge. A dose-ranging, placebo-controlled study of 86 patients used larazotide acetate (0.25, 1, 4, or 8 mg) or placebo 3 times per day with or without gluten challenge (2.4 g/d for 14 days).[60] The primary efficacy outcome was LA/MA ratio. However, LA/MA measurements were highly variable; it did not increase significantly following gluten challenge; and, among those receiving gluten challenge, the difference in the

LA/MA ratios for the larazotide acetate and placebo groups was not statistically significant. Nonetheless, larazotide acetate was associated with reduced gluten-induced gastrointestinal symptom severity. This effect was most evident at the lower dose levels, a phenomenon that was replicated in later studies.

A subsequent, larger gluten challenge study (2.7 g/d for 6 weeks) randomized 184 patients maintaining a GFD to larazotide acetate (1, 4, or 8 mg 3 times daily) or placebo.[61] Once again the primary efficacy outcome was not achieved because no significant differences in LA/MA ratios were observed. However, larazotide acetate at the lowest dose tested (1 mg) significantly reduced gluten-induced symptoms and, at the 1-mg and 4-mg doses, gluten-induced immune activation was inhibited, as shown by lower anti-TTG IgA levels.

More recently, results of a phase IIb clinical trial of larazotide acetate in 342 patients with nonresponsive CD, characterized by ongoing symptoms despite a GFD for 12 months or longer, were published.[62] Subjects were randomized to receive larazotide acetate (0.5, 1, or 2 mg 3 times daily) or placebo for 12 weeks. The primary efficacy outcome was improvement in the Celiac Disease Gastrointestinal Symptom Rating Scale (CeD-GSRS) score. This outcome was met for the lowest dose tested (0.5 mg) but not for the higher doses. Other benefits at the 0.5-mg dose were a decrease in patient-reported symptomatic days, a reduction in abdominal pain scores, and a decrease in the nongastrointestinal symptoms of headache and tiredness.

Given its excellent safety profile and its efficacy, at low dosage, in reducing symptoms in patients with nonresponsive CD, larazotide acetate is expected to move forward to a phase III registration study for this indication. Its mechanism of action in maintaining and restoring tight junction barrier function also make it an attractive agent for studies in other disorders characterized by increased intestinal permeability, including irritable bowel syndrome associated with diarrhea.

Tissue transglutaminase 2 inhibitors

Human transglutaminases (TGs) are multifunctional intracellular enzymes that play a crucial role in the pathogenesis of CD by catalyzing the deamidation of gluten peptide-bound glutamine residues, because of which their affinity for the HLA DQ2 and HLA DQ8 receptors increases. There are currently considered to be 3 classes of TG2 inhibitors that differ based on their mechanisms of action: competitive amine inhibitors, reversible inhibitors, and irreversible inhibitors. Competitive amine inhibitors inhibit TG2 activity by competing and blocking substrate access to the active site without covalently modifying the enzyme. A crosslink is formed between the natural glutamine substrate and the competitive amine inhibitor. The irreversible TG2 inhibitors link irreversibly with the enzyme by covalently modifying it. In a proof-of-concept study, Rauhavirta and colleagues[63] showed that the direct toxic effects (transepithelial resistance, cytoskeletal rearrangement, junction protein expression, and phosphorylation of extracellular signal–regulated kinase 1/2) of predigested gliadin on cultured intestinal epithelial Caco 2 cells were ameliorated by 2 inhibitors of TG2 (R281 and R283). Furthermore, the same investigators used an organ culture of small intestinal biopsies from patients with CD to measure secretion of TG2 autoantibodies into the culture medium and the densities of CD25-positive and IL-15–positive cells, Forkhead box protein 3 FOXP3-positive T_{regs}, and Ki-67–positive proliferating crypt cells following gluten exposure. The TG2 inhibitor R281 modified the gluten-induced increase in CD25-positive and IL-15–positive cells, T_{regs}, and crypt cell proliferation but had no effect on antibody secretion in biopsies from patients with CD. Even if these results are extremely promising, there are several potential side effects that nonselective TG inhibitors may exert, because the TG is a ubiquitous enzyme, and the amino acid sequence in the intestinal TG2 is similar to the one occurring in other human TGs. Therefore, the report of 3 highly soluble TG inhibitors (ZED1098, ZED1219, ZED1227) showing high selectivity for intestinal TG2 has suggested the possibility of their use in CD treatment. Nevertheless, developing an inhibitor that, after passing through the epithelial layer, could obtain at the lamina propria a sufficient concentration at the lowest possible systemic activity may be problematic. In addition, many gluten peptides are immunogenic, albeit at lower potency, without deamidation by TTG. Furthermore, TG2 deficiency is associated with the development of splenomegaly, autoantibodies, and immune complex glomerulonephritis in mice,[64] raising further concerns regarding the potential use of these inhibitors for the management of CD.

Human leukocyte antigen DQ2 blockers

The presentation of immunogenic oligopeptides on HLA-DQ2 or DQ8 by mucosal antigen-presenting cells to activate gliadin-specific T-cell responses is central to the pathogenesis of CD (see **Fig. 1**). Hence blockade of this pivotal event is an attractive target for CD therapy. To this end, immunogenic gliadin oligopeptides that interact with the binding groove of HLA-DQ2 have been analyzed to identify the most avid binders, and their amino acid compositions have been altered by substitution with natural and synthetic units to augment their binding affinity more than 50-fold with the goal of developing antagonistic analogues.[65] Such analogues can partially block T-cell activation and IFN-γ production by peripheral blood mononuclear cells from patients with CD exposed to native gliadin peptides in vitro. However, there are several challenges and limitations to this approach. The analogues may retain partial agonistic effects, may not completely block activation by native immunogenic peptides, or may not effectively access the key target antigen-presenting cells. There is also the potential for unwelcome immunosuppressive side effects of HLA blockade. Hence, inhibition of HLA-DQ2 remains in the preclinical development phase.

Antiinflammatory therapies

Being a chronic inflammatory disease, using steroidal antiinflammatory drugs or strategies targeting the involved cytokines, chemokines, and chemokine receptors has been considered for the treatment of nonresponsive or refractory CD. Understanding the involvement of individual inflammatory cytokines and chemokines (TNF-α, IFN-γ, IL-15, chemokine ligand 25 CCL25, and C-X-C motif chemokine 10 CXCL10) in the pathogenesis of CD as outlined in **Fig. 1** offers the opportunity to use biologic therapy in the treatment of this disease.

Glucocorticoids Glucocorticoids are generally reserved for nonresponsive or refractory CD or celiac crisis. Reports on the inhibitory effect of steroids on both B-cell and T-cell proliferation in in vitro studies or their effects on reduction of the lymphokine level released by the cultured cells indicated that they may be effective if given in addition to GFD to patients with active CD despite a GFD.[66] In a more recent study on 20 patients with CD, Ciacci and colleagues[67] showed a better clinical response in a group of patients treated with a combination of GFD and budesonide for 4 weeks compared with those treated with GFD alone. Budesonide is also routinely used in refractory CD type 1 even if its effectiveness to ameliorate inflammation not only in the distal ileum but also in the proximal small intestine (where most of the CD enteropathy occurs) has not been established.[68] In a proof-of-concept randomized controlled trial to test the effects of a short course of prednisolone along with GFD on the markers of apoptosis and antiapoptosis pathways in patients with CD, Shaliman and colleagues showed that although addition of prednisolone to GFD led to a significant reduction of apoptosis, it also led to decreases in epithelial cell regeneration. Systemic (eg, prednisone) or topical enteral (enteric-release budesonide) steroids seem to be very effective in the management of newly diagnosed, uncontrolled, and highly active CD presenting with the rare but serious complication of celiac crisis.[69]

Cytokines and chemokines

Anti–interferon gamma and anti–tumor necrosis factor alpha Based on the pathogenic role of IFN-γ and anti–TNF-α in CD (see **Fig. 1**), their blockade may prevent the activation of proteolytic matrix metalloproteinases and ultimately restore intestinal hemostasis.[70] IFN-γ–blocking antibodies seem to prevent damage of healthy intestinal mucosa exposed to the inflammatory cytokines released by gliadin-specific T-cell lines.[71] It has also been proposed that gliadin-induced IFN-γ secretion increases gliadin influx through the intestinal barrier and, therefore, the use of IFN-γ–blocking agents may also be effective by stopping this vicious cycle.[72] In anecdotal cases, monoclonal antibodies against TNF-α (infliximab) have been shown to be beneficial for patients with refractory CD not responding to steroid treatment.[73,74]

Anti–interleukin-15 IL-15 is secreted from the intestinal epithelium and antigen-presenting cells in response to gliadin peptides and plays an important role in the innate immune response in the intestinal mucosa of patients with CD. It induces the secretion of epithelial Major histocompatibility complex (MHC) class I chain-related protein A MICA, which binds to the NKG2D receptor located on the surface of IELs.[75] This ligand-receptor interaction is enhanced by IL-15, leading to stimulation and proliferation of cytotoxic T lymphocytes that induce epithelial apoptosis and also results in the development of refractory CD and its malignant transformation.[10] In transgenic mouse models overexpressing IL-15, with the consequent development of autoimmune enteropathy, blocking antibody against IL-15 was capable of efficiently reversing the intestinal damage.[76] IL-15 also prevents apoptosis of the cytotoxic IELs that play a central role in refractory CD via the JAK 3/STAT 5 signaling pathway. Therefore, anti–IL-15 human monoclonal antibody is a logical tool to treat refractory CD. These antibodies have been evaluated in patients affected by rheumatoid arthritis with disappointing results, and publication of exploratory studies in refractory CD are eagerly awaited.

Interleukin-10 IL-10 is an immunoregulatory cytokine in the intestinal tissue and suppresses inflammatory cytokine secretion from Th1 cells. Therefore, IL-10 is considered as a candidate for the treatment of Th1-mediated autoimmune disorders such as CD.[70] Although IL-10 was shown to suppress gliadin-induced T-cell activation in an ex vivo study of cultured intestinal biopsies for CD,[77] a pilot study on patients with refractory CD led to disappointing results, showing no pharmacologic efficacy.[78]

Lymphocytic recruitment blockade

Integrin α4β7 and mucosal addressin cell adhesion molecule-1 For migration and homing of lymphocytes to the intestinal mucosa, T cells express integrin ($\alpha_4\beta_7$), which is required for their binding to mucosal addressin cell adhesion molecule-1 (MAdCAM-1), located on intestinal vascular endothelial cells. Furthermore, natalizumab, a monoclonal antibody against α_4 integrin, and vedolizumab, a monoclonal antibody against $\alpha_4\beta_7$ integrin, have been shown to be effective in suppressing intestinal inflammation in patients with Crohn disease.[79] MAdCAM-1 has been shown to be significantly upregulated in treatment-naive patients with CD. Therefore, lymphocytic recruitment blockade using blockers of integrin $\alpha_4\beta_7$ and/or MAdCAM-1 are potential therapeutic targets for patients with CD.[80]

C-C chemokine receptor antagonists Eksteen and Adams[81] showed that the low-molecular-weight selective antagonist of the C-C chemokine receptor (CCR) for human chemokine CCL25 (GSK-1605786, CCX-282, Traficet-EN, ChemoCentryx, GlaxoSmithKline) selectively inhibits T-cell and B-cell entry into the small intestine while leaving the immune function at other anatomic sites unaffected in Crohn disease. Nevertheless, a similar study registered in clinicaltrials.gov targeting CD was completed in 2008 and its results have not been reported as yet.

Antigen-specific immunotherapy to induce tolerance to gluten

The inappropriate activation of immune responses to dietary gluten peptides is a primary defect in CD pathogenesis. CD is singular among autoimmune disorders in that the main environmental antigens responsible for initiating and perpetuating the harmful immune response are known and characterized. Hence, the induction of tolerance to these peptides represents an attractive opportunity for cure. This work in turn may lead to tolerance induction in other autoimmune diseases in which the environmental stimuli that drive disease activity are not yet defined.

Nexvax2 Antigen-specific desensitization is a leading therapy for allergic disorders and is believed to lead to the induction of $CD4^+$ T_{reg} cells that suppress antigen-responsive immune activation. A similar antigen-specific immunotherapy approach is being explored in CD using peptides that express leading gluten-associated antigenic epitopes administered by repeated injections at gradually increased dosages with the intention of achieving tolerance. The choice of peptide antigens used in Nexvax2 was guided by a broad, unbiased analysis of gluten-specific T cells in the peripheral blood of patients with CD during gluten challenge. Immunodominant peptides were identified, including 3 that mediated the activation of most of the gluten-specific T cells.[34]

In phase 1 studies, Nexvax2 was administered by intradermal injection to HLA-DQ2.5 genotype–positive patients with CD. Injection of the immunodominant peptides induced a gluten challenge–like reaction that included gastrointestinal symptoms and release of proinflammatory cytokines. Hence, the investigators introduced stepwise dose escalation (across a range from 3 µg to 900 µg over 9 weeks) that mitigated these reactions, particularly when a lower starting dose of 3 µg, in place of 30 µg, was implemented.[53]

Tolerizing immune modifying particles enveloping gliadin An alternative approach to antigen-specific immunotherapy uses tolerizing immune modifying particles (TIMP) composed of a biodegradable polymer poly(lactic-co-glycolic-acid) surface that envelops gliadin in its core (TIMP-GLI). The nanoparticles are thought to traffic to lymphoid tissues, including the spleen, and release their cargo in an environment in which tolerizing antigen-presenting cells are predominant.[82] The safety and pharmacokinetic profile of intravenous TIMP-GLIA are being evaluated in a phase 1 clinical trial in subjects with treated CD (NCT03486990).

SUMMARY

A lifelong, strict GFD is a highly effective treatment of many patients with CD. However, the GFD is often both challenging and burdensome. Moreover, a substantial minority of patients with CD develop nonresponsive or refractory CD with persisting symptoms and mucosal injury despite their best attempts to follow a GFD. Hence there is a clear major unmet medical need for therapies to augment dietary gluten avoidance. The current knowledge of the sequential steps in CD pathogenesis has revealed multiple potential therapeutic targets for research and drug development. Attractive options that have been explored include enzymatic gluten degradation either before or after food ingestion, binding and sequestration of gluten in the gastro-intestinal lumen, restoration of epithelial tight junction barrier function, inhibition of TTG-mediated potentiation of gliadin oligopeptide immunogenicity or of HLA-mediated gliadin presentation, and induction of tolerance to gluten, as well as a diverse array of antiinflammatory interventions to reduce mucosal inflammation and injury. As yet, there is no approved pharmacologic therapy for CD. It is likely that initial approved treatments will act as adjuvants to the GFD for treatment of nonresponsive or refractory CD. However, it is hoped that subsequent developments will include agents to avoid the harmful effects of occasional inadvertent dietary gluten contamination and to ease the burden of attempting to following a lifelong, continuous GFD. The ultimate goal for nondietary therapies in CD is to allow patients to resume a normal diet through induction of tolerance to ingested gluten peptides. This life-changing advance for patients with CD could also act as a pivotal event in the prevention and management of other autoimmune disorders for which the environmental activators of disease are not well characterized.

REFERENCES

1. Fasano A, Catassi C. Clinical practice. Celiac disease. N Engl J Med 2012; 367(25):2419–26.
2. Malamut G, Cellier C. Refractory celiac disease. Expert Rev Gastroenterol Hepatol 2014;8(3):323–8.
3. Shah S, Akbari M, Vanga R, et al. Patient perception of treatment burden is high in celiac disease compared with other common conditions. Am J Gastroenterol 2014;109(9):1304–11.
4. Vanga RR, Kelly CP. Novel therapeutic approaches for celiac disease. Discov Med 2014;17(95):285–93.
5. Leonard MM, Serena G, Sturgeon C, et al. Genetics and celiac disease: the importance of screening. Expert Rev Gastroenterol Hepatol 2015;9(2):209–15.
6. Fasano A. Zonulin and its regulation of intestinal barrier function: the biological door to inflammation, autoimmunity, and cancer. Physiol Rev 2011;91(1):151–75.
7. Reinke Y, Zimmer KP, Naim HY. Toxic peptides in Frazer's fraction interact with the actin cytoskeleton and affect the targeting and function of intestinal proteins. Exp Cell Res 2009;315(19):3442–52.
8. Lammers KM, Lu R, Brownley J, et al. Gliadin induces an increase in intestinal permeability and zonulin release by binding to the chemokine receptor CXCR3. Gastroenterology 2008;135(1):194–204.e3.
9. Harris KM, Fasano A, Mann DL. Monocytes differentiated with IL-15 support Th17 and Th1 responses to wheat gliadin: implications for celiac disease. Clin Immunol 2010;135(3):430–9.
10. Mention JJ, Ben Ahmed M, Begue B, et al. Interleukin 15: a key to disrupted intra-epithelial lymphocyte homeostasis and lymphomagenesis in celiac disease. Gastroenterology 2003;125(3):730–45.
11. Kim SM, Mayassi T, Jabri B. Innate immunity: actuating the gears of celiac disease pathogenesis. Best Pract Res Clin Gastroenterol 2015;29(3):425–35.
12. Diosdado B, van Bakel H, Strengman E, et al. Neutrophil recruitment and barrier impairment in celiac disease: a genomic study. Clin Gastroenterol Hepatol 2007; 5(5):574–81.
13. Lammers KM, Khandelwal S, Chaudhry F, et al. Identification of a novel immuno-modulatory gliadin peptide that causes interleukin-8 release in a chemokine

receptor CXCR3-dependent manner only in patients with coeliac disease. Immunology 2011;132(3):432–40.

14. Lammers KM, Chieppa M, Liu L, et al. Gliadin induces neutrophil migration via engagement of the formyl peptide receptor, FPR1. PLoS One 2015;10(9): e0138338.

15. Lammers KM, Herrera MG, Dodero VI. Translational chemistry meets gluten-related disorders. ChemistryOpen 2018;7(3):217–32.

16. Marafini I, Monteleone I, Di Fusco D, et al. TNF-alpha producing innate lymphoid cells (ILCs) are increased in active celiac disease and contribute to promote intestinal atrophy in mice. PLoS One 2015;10(5):e0126291.

17. Jabri B, Sollid LM. T cells in celiac disease. J Immunol 2017;198(8):3005–14.

18. Rubio-Tapia A, Murray JA. Celiac disease. Curr Opin Gastroenterol 2010;26(2): 116–22.

19. Sapone A, Lammers KM, Mazzarella G, et al. Differential mucosal IL-17 expression in two gliadin-induced disorders: gluten sensitivity and the autoimmune enteropathy celiac disease. Int Arch Allergy Immunol 2010;152(1):75–80.

20. Granzotto M, dal Bo S, Quaglia S, et al. Regulatory T-cell function is impaired in celiac disease. Dig Dis Sci 2009;54(7):1513–9.

21. Serena G, Yan S, Camhi S, et al. Proinflammatory cytokine interferon-gamma and microbiome-derived metabolites dictate epigenetic switch between forkhead box protein 3 isoforms in coeliac disease. Clin Exp Immunol 2017; 187(3):490–506.

22. Senger S, Sapone A, Fiorentino MR, et al. Celiac disease histopathology recapitulates Hedgehog downregulation, consistent with wound healing processes activation. PLoS One 2015;10(12):e0144634.

23. Martin VJ, Leonard MM, Fiechtner L, et al. Transitioning from descriptive to mechanistic understanding of the microbiome: the need for a prospective longitudinal approach to predicting disease. J Pediatr 2016;179:240–8.

24. Wacklin P, Kaukinen K, Tuovinen E, et al. The duodenal microbiota composition of adult celiac disease patients is associated with the clinical manifestation of the disease. Inflamm Bowel Dis 2013;19(5):934–41.

25. Tjellstrom B, Hogberg L, Stenhammar L, et al. Faecal short-chain fatty acid pattern in childhood coeliac disease is normalised after more than one year's gluten-free diet. Microb Ecol Health Dis 2013;24. https://doi.org/10.3402/mehd. v24i0.20905.

26. Nistal E, Caminero A, Herran AR, et al. Differences of small intestinal bacteria populations in adults and children with/without celiac disease: effect of age, gluten diet, and disease. Inflamm Bowel Dis 2012;18(4):649–56.

27. Collado MC, Donat E, Ribes-Koninckx C, et al. Specific duodenal and faecal bacterial groups associated with paediatric coeliac disease. J Clin Pathol 2009;62(3): 264–9.

28. Ou G, Hedberg M, Horstedt P, et al. Proximal small intestinal microbiota and identification of rod-shaped bacteria associated with childhood celiac disease. Am J Gastroenterol 2009;104(12):3058–67.

29. Nadal I, Donat E, Ribes-Koninckx C, et al. Imbalance in the composition of the duodenal microbiota of children with coeliac disease. J Med Microbiol 2007; 56(Pt 12):1669–74.

30. Meisel M, Mayassi T, Fehlner-Peach H, et al. Interleukin-15 promotes intestinal dysbiosis with butyrate deficiency associated with increased susceptibility to colitis. ISME J 2017;11(1):15–30.

31. Janssen G, Christis C, Kooy-Winkelaar Y, et al. Ineffective degradation of immunogenic gluten epitopes by currently available digestive enzyme supplements. PLoS One 2015;10(6):e0128065.
32. Krishnareddy S, Stier K, Recanati M, et al. Commercially available glutenases: a potential hazard in coeliac disease. Therap Adv Gastroenterol 2017;10(6): 473–81.
33. Siegel M, Garber ME, Spencer AG, et al. Safety, tolerability, and activity of ALV003: results from two phase 1 single, escalating-dose clinical trials. Dig Dis Sci 2012;57(2):440–50.
34. Tye-Din JA, Anderson RP, Ffrench RA, et al. The effects of ALV003 pre-digestion of gluten on immune response and symptoms in celiac disease in vivo. Clin Immunol 2010;134(3):289–95.
35. Lahdeaho ML, Kaukinen K, Laurila K, et al. Glutenase ALV003 attenuates gluten-induced mucosal injury in patients with celiac disease. Gastroenterology 2014; 146(7):1649–58.
36. Murray JA, Kelly CP, Green PHR, et al, CeliAction Study Group of I. No difference between latiglutenase and placebo in reducing villus atrophy or improving symptoms in patients with symptomatic celiac disease. Gastroenterology 2017;152(4): 787–98.e2.
37. Al-Bawardy B, Barlow JM, Vasconcelos RN, et al. Cross-sectional imaging in refractory celiac disease. Abdom Radiol (NY) 2017;42(2):389–95.
38. Pyle GG, Paaso B, Anderson BE, et al. Effect of pretreatment of food gluten with prolyl endopeptidase on gluten-induced malabsorption in celiac sprue. Clin Gastroenterol Hepatol 2005;3(7):687–94.
39. Stepniak D, Spaenij-Dekking L, Mitea C, et al. Highly efficient gluten degradation with a newly identified prolyl endoprotease: implications for celiac disease. Am J Physiol Gastrointest Liver Physiol 2006;291(4):G621–9.
40. Mitea C, Havenaar R, Drijfhout JW, et al. Efficient degradation of gluten by a prolyl endoprotease in a gastrointestinal model: implications for coeliac disease. Gut 2008;57(1):25–32.
41. Gordon SR, Stanley EJ, Wolf S, et al. Computational design of an alpha-gliadin peptidase. J Am Chem Soc 2012;134(50):20513–20.
42. Wolf C, Siegel JB, Tinberg C, et al. Engineering of Kuma030: a gliadin peptidase that rapidly degrades immunogenic gliadin peptides in gastric conditions. J Am Chem Soc 2015;137(40):13106–13.
43. Pinier M, Fuhrmann G, Galipeau HJ, et al. The copolymer P(HEMA-co-SS) binds gluten and reduces immune response in gluten-sensitized mice and human tissues. Gastroenterology 2012;142(2):316–25.e1-12.
44. Warny M, Fatimi A, Bostwick EF, et al. Bovine immunoglobulin concentrate-*Clostridium difficile* retains *C difficile* toxin neutralising activity after passage through the human stomach and small intestine. Gut 1999;44(2):212–7.
45. Gujral N, Lobenberg R, Suresh M, et al. In-vitro and in-vivo binding activity of chicken egg yolk immunoglobulin Y (IgY) against gliadin in food matrix. J Agric Food Chem 2012;60(12):3166–72.
46. Gujral N, Suh JW, Sunwoo HH. Effect of anti-gliadin IgY antibody on epithelial intestinal integrity and inflammatory response induced by gliadin. BMC Immunol 2015;16:41.
47. Di Cagno R, De Angelis M, Auricchio S, et al. Sourdough bread made from wheat and nontoxic flours and started with selected lactobacilli is tolerated in celiac sprue patients. Appl Environ Microbiol 2004;70(2):1088–96.

48. Rizzello CG, De Angelis M, Di Cagno R, et al. Highly efficient gluten degradation by lactobacilli and fungal proteases during food processing: new perspectives for celiac disease. Appl Environ Microbiol 2007;73(14):4499–507.
49. Di Cagno R, Barbato M, Di Camillo C, et al. Gluten-free sourdough wheat baked goods appear safe for young celiac patients: a pilot study. J Pediatr Gastroenterol Nutr 2010;51(6):777–83.
50. Greco L, Gobbetti M, Auricchio R, et al. Safety for patients with celiac disease of baked goods made of wheat flour hydrolyzed during food processing. Clin Gastroenterol Hepatol 2011;9(1):24–9.
51. De Angelis M, Rizzello CG, Fasano A, et al. VSL#3 probiotic preparation has the capacity to hydrolyze gliadin polypeptides responsible for celiac sprue. Biochim Biophys Acta 2006;1762(1):80–93.
52. Madsen K, Cornish A, Soper P, et al. Probiotic bacteria enhance murine and human intestinal epithelial barrier function. Gastroenterology 2001;121(3):580–91.
53. Daveson AJ, Jones DM, Gaze S, et al. Effect of hookworm infection on wheat challenge in celiac disease–a randomised double-blinded placebo controlled trial. PLoS One 2011;6(3):e17366.
54. Fasano A. Regulation of intercellular tight junctions by zonula occludens toxin and its eukaryotic analogue zonulin. Ann N Y Acad Sci 2000;915:214–22.
55. Drago S, El Asmar R, Di Pierro M, et al. Gliadin, zonulin and gut permeability: effects on celiac and non-celiac intestinal mucosa and intestinal cell lines. Scand J Gastroenterol 2006;41(4):408–19.
56. Duerksen DR, Wilhelm-Boyles C, Veitch R, et al. A comparison of antibody testing, permeability testing, and zonulin levels with small-bowel biopsy in celiac disease patients on a gluten-free diet. Dig Dis Sci 2010;55(4):1026–31.
57. Gopalakrishnan S, Durai M, Kitchens K, et al. Larazotide acetate regulates epithelial tight junctions in vitro and in vivo. Peptides 2012;35(1):86–94.
58. Gopalakrishnan S, Tripathi A, Tamiz AP, et al. Larazotide acetate promotes tight junction assembly in epithelial cells. Peptides 2012;35(1):95–101.
59. Paterson BM, Lammers KM, Arrieta MC, et al. The safety, tolerance, pharmacokinetic and pharmacodynamic effects of single doses of AT-1001 in coeliac disease subjects: a proof of concept study. Aliment Pharmacol Ther 2007;26(5):757–66.
60. Leffler DA, Kelly CP, Abdallah HZ, et al. A randomized, double-blind study of larazotide acetate to prevent the activation of celiac disease during gluten challenge. Am J Gastroenterol 2012;107(10):1554–62.
61. Kelly CP, Green PH, Murray JA, et al, Larazotide Acetate Celiac Disease Study Group. Larazotide acetate in patients with coeliac disease undergoing a gluten challenge: a randomised placebo-controlled study. Aliment Pharmacol Ther 2013;37(2):252–62.
62. Leffler DA, Kelly CP, Green PH, et al. Larazotide acetate for persistent symptoms of celiac disease despite a gluten-free diet: a randomized controlled trial. Gastroenterology 2015;148(7):1311–1319 e6.
63. Rauhavirta T, Oittinen M, Kivisto R, et al. Are transglutaminase 2 inhibitors able to reduce gliadin-induced toxicity related to celiac disease? A proof-of-concept study. J Clin Immunol 2013;33(1):134–42.
64. Szondy Z, Sarang Z, Molnar P, et al. Transglutaminase 2-/- mice reveal a phagocytosis-associated crosstalk between macrophages and apoptotic cells. Proc Natl Acad Sci U S A 2003;100(13):7812–7.
65. Kapoerchan VV, Wiesner M, Hillaert U, et al. Design, synthesis and evaluation of high-affinity binders for the celiac disease associated HLA-DQ2 molecule. Mol Immunol 2010;47(5):1091–7.

66. Wahl SM, Wilton JM, Rosenstreich DL, et al. The role of macrophages in the production of lymphokines by T and B lymphocytes. J Immunol 1975;114(4): 1296–301.
67. Ciacci C, Citterio B, Betti M, et al. Functional differential immune responses of *Mytilus galloprovincialis* to bacterial challenge. Comp Biochem Physiol B Biochem Mol Biol 2009;153(4):365–71.
68. Bakshi A, Stephen S, Borum ML, et al. Emerging therapeutic options for celiac disease: potential alternatives to a gluten-free diet. Gastroenterol Hepatol (N Y) 2012;8(9):582–8.
69. Jamma S, Rubio-Tapia A, Kelly CP, et al. Celiac crisis is a rare but serious complication of celiac disease in adults. Clin Gastroenterol Hepatol 2010;8(7):587–90.
70. Schuppan D, Junker Y, Barisani D. Celiac disease: from pathogenesis to novel therapies. Gastroenterology 2009;137(6):1912–33.
71. Przemioslo RT, Lundin KE, Sollid LM, et al. Histological changes in small bowel mucosa induced by gliadin sensitive T lymphocytes can be blocked by anti-interferon gamma antibody. Gut 1995;36(6):874–9.
72. Bethune MT, Siegel M, Howles-Banerji S, et al. Interferon-gamma released by gluten-stimulated celiac disease-specific intestinal T cells enhances the transepithelial flux of gluten peptides. J Pharmacol Exp Ther 2009;329(2):657–68.
73. Gillett HR, Arnott ID, McIntyre M, et al. Successful infliximab treatment for steroid-refractory celiac disease: a case report. Gastroenterology 2002;122(3):800–5.
74. Costantino G, della Torre A, Lo Presti MA, et al. Treatment of life-threatening type I refractory coeliac disease with long-term infliximab. Dig Liver Dis 2008;40(1): 74–7.
75. Maiuri L, Ciacci C, Auricchio S, et al. Interleukin 15 mediates epithelial changes in celiac disease. Gastroenterology 2000;119(4):996–1006.
76. Yokoyama S, Watanabe N, Sato N, et al. Antibody-mediated blockade of IL-15 reverses the autoimmune intestinal damage in transgenic mice that overexpress IL-15 in enterocytes. Proc Natl Acad Sci U S A 2009;106(37):15849–54.
77. Salvati VM, Mazzarella G, Gianfrani C, et al. Recombinant human interleukin 10 suppresses gliadin dependent T cell activation in ex vivo cultured coeliac intestinal mucosa. Gut 2005;54(1):46–53.
78. van Belzen MJ, Mulder CJ, Pearson PL, et al. The tissue transglutaminase gene is not a primary factor predisposing to celiac disease. Am J Gastroenterol 2001; 96(12):3337–40.
79. Ghosh S, Goldin E, Gordon FH, et al. Natalizumab for active Crohn's disease. N Engl J Med 2003;348(1):24–32.
80. Di Sabatino A, Rovedatti L, Rosado MM, et al. Increased expression of mucosal addressin cell adhesion molecule 1 in the duodenum of patients with active celiac disease is associated with depletion of integrin alpha4beta7-positive T cells in blood. Hum Pathol 2009;40(5):699–704.
81. Eksteen B, Adams DH. GSK-1605786, a selective small-molecule antagonist of the CCR9 chemokine receptor for the treatment of Crohn's disease. IDrugs 2010;13(7):472–81.
82. Getts DR, Turley DM, Smith CE, et al. Tolerance induced by apoptotic antigen-coupled leukocytes is induced by PD-L1+ and IL-10-producing splenic macrophages and maintained by T regulatory cells. J Immunol 2011;187(5):2405–17.

Nonceliac Wheat Sensitivity

An Immune-Mediated Condition with Systemic Manifestations

Umberto Volta, MD[a], Roberto De Giorgio, MD[b],
Giacomo Caio, MD[a,c], Melanie Uhde, PhD[d,e],
Roberto Manfredini, MD[b], Armin Alaedini, PhD[d,e,f],*

KEYWORDS

- Wheat • Systemic immune activation • Intestinal barrier function • Gluten
- Amylase/protease inhibitor • Fructan • Biomarkers • Antibody to native gliadin

KEY POINTS

- Nonceliac wheat sensitivity (NCWS) is a condition characterized by intestinal and extraintestinal symptoms that occur after the ingestion of wheat and related cereals in patients without celiac disease or wheat allergy.
- Recent findings provide a biological basis for NCWS, revealing a state of systemic immune activation in conjunction with a compromised intestinal epithelium in a significant subset of affected individuals.
- The pathogenesis of NCWS is likely to be the result of a complex interplay among different factors, including specific components of wheat and related cereals, intestinal barrier function, gut microbiota, and innate and adaptive immunity.
- NCWS can present at any age, but its frequency appears to be higher in young adults (3rd- 4th decades of life) and in females.
- Currently, a double-blind placebo-controlled crossover trial is the only widely accepted method to confirm NCWS, although research is underway to establish biomarkers to aid the diagnosis.

Disclosure: The authors declare no competing interests.
Funded by: National Center for Advancing Translational Sciences, NIH. Grant number(s): UL1 TR000040.
^a Department of Medical and Surgical Sciences, St. Orsola-Malpighi Hospital, University of Bologna, Via Zamboni, 33, Bologna BO 40126, Italy; ^b Department of Medical Sciences, Nuovo Arcispedale St. Anna in Cona, University of Ferrara, Via Savonarola, 9, Ferrara FE 44121, Italy; ^c Mucosal Immunology and Biology Research Center, Building 114 16th Street, Charlestown, MA 02129, USA; ^d Department of Medicine, Columbia University Medical Center, 1130 Saint Nicholas Avenue, New York, NY 10032, USA; ^e Celiac Disease Center, Columbia University Medical Center, 180 Fort Washington Avenue, New York, NY 10032, USA; ^f Institute of Human Nutrition, Columbia University Medical Center, 630 West 168th Street, New York, NY 10032, USA
* Corresponding author. Department of Medicine, Columbia University Medical Center, 630 West 168th Street, New York, NY 10032.
E-mail address: aa819@columbia.edu

INTRODUCTION

Over the past two decades, the incidence of diseases believed to be induced by the ingestion of wheat and related gluten-containing cereals, including rye and barley, has increased.[1] This trend seems to be caused by not only a significant improvement in diagnostic tools,[2,3] but also indicates an actual increase in disease incidence.[4] The reasons for such a rise are not entirely clear. Improved hygiene, exposure to certain infectious agents, gut microbial dysbiosis resulting from the use of antibiotics or other drugs and the changing dietary habits, and alterations in the cultivation, preparation, and processing of gluten-containing cereals have been researched or discussed in this context, but firm conclusions have not been reached.[3]

This background sets the basis for discussing a much-debated condition within the scientific community, and in particular, among experts gathered in four recent consensus conferences held in London, Munich, Salerno, and Merano from 2011 to 2016.[5–8] Distinct from celiac disease (CD) (and its primary related autoimmune disorder, dermatitis herpetiformis) and wheat allergy, a new condition has been identified and referred to as nonceliac gluten sensitivity or nonceliac wheat sensitivity (NCWS), a term that has been coined primarily to distinguish the condition from the clinically overlapping CD. NCWS Is now recognized as a condition triggered by an adverse reaction to certain wheat components and characterized by gastrointestinal, namely irritable bowel syndrome (IBS)-like, symptoms, and by extraintestinal manifestations, occurring a few hours or days after the ingestion of foods made with gluten-containing cereals (ie, wheat, rye, or barley). The associated symptoms improve with the withdrawal of the offending cereals and relapse after rechallenge. Exclusion of both CD and wheat allergy by established tests is a requirement for suspecting NCWS in patients on a gluten-containing diet. Although gluten has been the chief suspect as the triggering component of symptoms in NCWS, other components of wheat and related cereals may also be involved in symptom generation, either solely or possibly in conjunction with gluten.[5–8] Growing interest has been devoted to a group of α-amylase/protease inhibitors, commonly referred to as amylase/trypsin inhibitors (ATIs), and to the so-called fermentable oligosaccharides, disaccharides, monosaccharides, and polyols (FODMAPs).[9,10] As such, NCWS may be etiologically heterogeneous as clinically characterized currently, with subsets of patients responding to different components of wheat and related cereals. The diagnosis of NCWS relies on clinical criteria because of the lack of established biomarkers, making the diagnosis of this condition a clinical challenge.[5–8] Self-diagnosed NCWS may also be attributable to a placebo effect in a subset of individuals.[11,12] However, the use of validated questionnaires has been shown to be helpful in assessing the symptom variation before and after the exclusion of gluten-containing cereals, thus allowing the identification of patients with true NCWS.[7] Although inconvenient in daily practice, a double-blind, placebo-controlled crossover trial (DBPCC) is a particularly useful tool to establish and confirm the diagnosis.[7,8] Regardless of the apparently normal villus architecture, as detected by current technology and methods, a significant proportion of patients with NCWS seems to display mild intestinal malabsorption resulting in low levels of vitamin D_3, ferritin, and folic acid.[13] The mechanism leading to selective malabsorption is likely related to inflammatory changes in the small intestinal mucosa caused by innate immune activation, epithelial barrier impairment, and possible deleterious changes in the gut microbial population.[14] Recent research suggests that a combination of serologic markers of immune activation and intestinal cell damage may have utility in aiding the diagnosis of the condition in the near future.[15]

Because of the inadequate level of knowledge about the condition and the unmet needs in clinical practice, the present review aims to provide physicians with a thorough account and practical indications related to various aspects concerning NCWS, including pathogenesis, clinical picture, diagnosis, treatment, and future directions for research.

PATHOGENIC MECHANISMS

The pathogenesis of NCWS is likely to be multifactorial, with the innate immune response playing a key role. Several studies have identified an altered expression of innate immune components in response to wheat consumption in heterogeneous cohorts of wheat-sensitive individuals, including mucosal toll-like receptor 2,[16,17] peripheral blood mononuclear cells–derived interleukin-10, granulocyte colony–stimulating factor, transforming growth factor-α, and the chemokine CXCL-10.[18–20] Although wheat-sensitive individuals lack a significant increase in intraepithelial lymphocyte (IEL) infiltration, a characteristic histology in CD, an elevated frequency of interferon-γ-producing type 1 innate lymphoid cells in the rectal mucosa after oral wheat challenge has been shown in NCWS patients.[21] In line with these findings, increased mRNA levels of interferon-γ have been detected in the mucosal tissue of NCWS patients on gluten challenge.[22] However, it is not clear whether the increased interleukin-10 mRNA levels are mediated by the activation of innate or adaptive immune cells. The production of gliadin-specific antibodies in wheat-sensitive individuals[15,23,24] is suggestive of a concomitant activation of the adaptive immune response in NCWS, although the lack of CD-specific markers (anti–tissue transglutaminase antibodies and anti–deamidated gliadin antibodies) points to a mechanism that is significantly different from that in CD.

An impaired intestinal epithelial barrier has also been demonstrated *in vivo* (by lactulose-mannitol test) and *ex vivo* (altered tight junction protein expression on colonic mucosal biopsies) in a subset of patients exhibiting HLA-DQ2/DQ8 haplotypes and in whom wheat-evoked IBS-like symptoms is found.[18] Other data supporting the so-called "leaky gut" aspect in the context of NCWS include increased duodenal myosin light chain kinase activity and elevated colonocyte claudin-15 expression.[25] Notably, these alterations were reversible in NCWS patients after the withdrawal of gluten-containing food and were accompanied by symptom remission. In addition, intestinal dysbiosis might contribute to epithelial barrier dysfunction and associated inflammatory response to gluten, thereby contributing to the pathogenesis of NCWS, similarly to what has been shown in other disorders, such as CD, IBS, and inflammatory bowel disease.[26–29]

A recent study by Uhde and colleagues[15] has provided compelling evidence for the existence of a compromised intestinal barrier in a well-defined cohort of NCWS patients that results in a systemic immune response to microbial and dietary antigens. Serum levels of lipopolysaccharide (LPS)-binding proteins (sCD14 and LPS binding protein) and antibody reactivity to microbial products (LPS, flagellin) were found to be elevated in patients with NCWS, and to correlate with circulating levels of intestinal fatty acid-binding protein (FABP2), suggesting a compromised gut barrier and microbial translocation. On the introduction of a diet free of wheat and related cereals, the increase in markers of immune activation and epithelial cell damage changed significantly toward normalization in affected individuals, demonstrating a link between wheat-containing diet, a dysfunctional intestinal barrier, and systemic immune activation as underlying mechanistic components in NCWS. These results have demonstrated the presence of objective markers of systemic immune activation and gut epithelial cell damage in individuals who report sensitivity to wheat in the absence of CD, providing a biologic basis to explain the intestinal and extraintestinal manifestations of condition.[15] The presumed sequence of events leading to the systemic immune activation and associated symptoms in NCWS, as suggested by these data, is shown in **Fig. 1**.

CLINICAL PICTURE

Epidemiologic data on NCWS are not available because the diagnosis of this condition is still uncertain due to lack of biomarkers. Depending on the clinical setting, the prevalence of NCWS has been suggested to vary from 0.6% in primary care to 6% in tertiary care,[5,30] whereas in a multicenter study, the observed prevalence was 3.2% among more than 12.000 patients examined in 38 tertiary care centers.[31] This survey showed that NCWS was much more prevalent in young adult women than in men

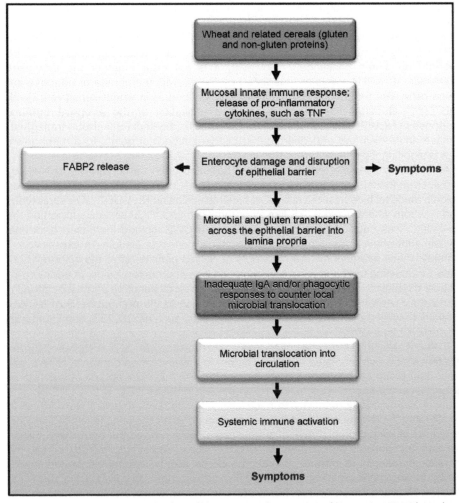

Fig. 1. Diagrammatic representation of the proposed sequence of events in NCWS based on the available data. TNF, tumor necrosis factor.

(female to male ratio = 5:1; mean age, 38 years), and rare in childhood and elderly. The study also found a similar frequency for NCWS and CD (NCWS/CD = 1.14). The clinical presentation of NCWS resembles IBS, although extraintestinal manifestations may be substantially more prevalent in NCWS.[16,31] Symptoms occur after a few hours to days following the ingestion of wheat and related cereals (ie, gluten-containing foods), and usually dissipate relatively rapidly after the withdrawal of the offending foods, and return soon after challenge. Before establishing NCWS, patients should be tested for CD serology and specific IgE antibodies to wheat allergens to rule out CD and wheat allergy while they are still on a gluten/wheat-containing diet.[7-10] Patients with NCWS have been reported to complain of gastrointestinal symptoms, such as bloating and abdominal pain, in more than 80% of cases.[31] Diarrhea is reported by about half of cases, whereas 20% to 30% of NCWS patients complain of alternating bowel and even constipation.[31] Other manifestations affecting the gastrointestinal tract, such as gastroesophageal reflux disease, nausea, vomiting, aerophagia, and aphthous stomatitis, are reported by 30% to 50% of NCWS patients.[7,16] The extraintestinal manifestations in NCWS encompass a broad spectrum of symptoms, among which fatigue, headache, anxiety, and cognitive difficulties feature prominently, affecting some 30% to 50% of patients.[31,32] Fibromyalgia-like symptoms, including diffuse and migratory joint and muscle pain, were observed in up to 30% of cases.[33] Although manifestations of presumed neurologic[32] and rheumatologic[33] origin can also be detected in IBS, skin complaints seem to be more specific to NCWS.[34] Skin rash and dermatitis have been found to be reported by up to 30% of patients.[31,34] Regarding laboratory abnormalities in NCWS patients, malabsorption features, such as low levels of vitamin D_3 (up to 16%) leading to osteopenia,[35] ferritin (up to 23%), and folic acid (up to 11%), which can be because of small intestinal microinflammation, have been reported.[13] About one-fifth of NCWS patients have been reported to have a family history of CD.[31,36,37] Based on these data, serologic screening for CD may be recommended in first-degree relatives of NCWS patients. Similarly to IBS, a large proportion of NCWS patients displays lactose and, less frequently, fructose intolerance.[31] About 20% of NCWS patients are positive for IgE antibodies to inhalants and foods including mites, graminaceae, shellfish, and other alimentary molecules.[31] In line with these findings, a subset of NCWS patients may complain of multiple food hypersensitivities, including food antigens other than those from wheat and related cereals.[38] In contrast with initial studies that ruled out an association between NCWS and autoimmunity,[17] more recent data point to a high prevalence of autoimmune markers (antinuclear antibodies) and autoimmune disorders (mainly Hashimoto thyroiditis) among NCWS patients (**Table 1**).[39,40] In contrast to CD, current data do not point to an association between NCWS and the development of complications, such as small intestinal lymphoma, small bowel adenocarcinoma, and ulcerative jejunoileitis.[4-8]

DIAGNOSTIC CRITERIA

Significant effort has been directed at identifying specific criteria for NCWS diagnosis. Earlier in this effort, the diagnostic approach relied only on exclusion criteria because symptomatic patients were labeled as NCWS after the exclusion of CD (ie, absence of anti–tissue transglutaminase/endomysial antibodies and of villus atrophy)[41] and wheat allergy (ie, negative serum IgE antibodies to wheat allergens and relevant skin prick tests).[42] Although the exclusion of these two disorders remains a mandatory prerequisite, during the third Consensus Conference on NCWS, a panel of experts made a significant step forward by introducing positive criteria, including (1) the evaluation

Table 1
Immunologic, genetic, and histopathologic features in NCWS patients

References	Antibodies to Native Gliadin (%)	HLA-DQ2/DQ8 (%)	Marsh 1 at Duodenal Biopsy (%)	Antinuclear Antibodies (%)	Autoimmune Disorders (%)	CD Family History (%)
Sapone et al,[17] 2011	48	46	84	—	—	—
Carroccio et al,[24] 2012; Carroccio et al,[39] 2015	50	75	96	46	29	14
Francavilla et al,[43]	66	46	26	—	—	—
Aziz et al,[36]	—	53	—	—	10	12
Kabbani et al,[37]	—	42	—	—	12	13
Volta et al,[23] 2012; Volta et al,[31] 2014; Volta et al,[40] 2016	56	46	46	37	14	18

Antibodies to native gluten, genetic haplotype, duodenal histology, autoimmune features, and familiarity for celiac disease in patients with nonceliac wheat sensitivity. Marsh 1 is intraepithelial lymphocytes >25/100 epithelial cells at high-power field.

of symptoms before and after gluten/wheat exclusion from the diet by means of a modified version of the Gastrointestinal Symptom Rating Scale (GSRS) integrated with extraintestinal manifestations, (2) the identification of potential biomarkers, and (3) the standardization of DBPCC for confirming the diagnosis.[7] The first step of the diagnostic work-up for NCWS is based on the symptom assessment (scored from 1 as very mild to 10 as very severe) at baseline (when patients are still on a gluten/wheat-containing diet) and weekly for 6 weeks on gluten-free diet (GFD) by using the modified GSRS questionnaire.[7] A GFD-dependent symptom decrease of greater than 30% compared with baseline in at least three symptoms is regarded as a criterion to suspect NCWS.

The identification of established biomarkers for NCWS is still eagerly awaited. Several studies have reported elevated IgG antigluten antibodies (AGA) in more than half of NCWS patients (see **Table 1**),[23,24,43] although these antibodies lack specificity for NCWS, being also found in CD, certain other autoimmune disorders, and some apparently healthy subjects.[44] Nonetheless, their detection in symptomatic patients may support the diagnosis of NCWS.[45] The diagnostic potential of antibody reactivity to gluten as a possible biomarker of NCWS has been recently expanded by the finding of increased levels of the IgM class AGA in the sera of NCWS patients in comparison with healthy individuals.[15]

A series of intestinal cell damage and systemic immune activation markers has been recently described as having the potential to identify NCWS.[15] Serum levels of sCD14 and LPS-binding protein, both related to acute-phase innate immune response to bacterial components, and antibody reactivity to bacterial antigens, have been found to be significantly increased in NCWS, suggesting systemic immune activation in response to microbial translocation. In addition, serum levels of FABP2, a marker of increased intestinal epithelial cell injury and turnover rate, was shown to be elevated in NCWS compared with control subjects, pointing to a compromised intestinal barrier against antigen translocation from the gut lumen. Of particular significance, all of the aforementioned biomarkers decreased significantly toward normalization after the exclusion of wheat and related cereals from diet, which was associated with improvement in symptoms. Although no single biomarker is considered diagnostic, the principal component analysis of the previously mentioned biomarkers, including various antibody isotype reactivity to gluten, allowed for the differentiation of NCWS individuals from CD and healthy control subjects.[15,46] The data establish the presence of objective markers of systemic immune activation and epithelial cell damage in NCWS, suggesting that a combination of biomarkers may have utility for identifying patients or specific patient subsets. A recent study used these same markers to identify a significant subset of patients with myalgic encephalomyelitis/chronic fatigue syndrome and gastrointestinal symptoms as potentially having NCWS.[47]

Another interesting aid in the diagnosis of NCWS might be the chemokine (CXCL10). In children and adults with suspected NCWS, the *in vitro* stimulation of peripheral blood mononuclear cells by wheat extracts (Manitoba) resulted in significantly increased secretion of this chemokine, which was undetectable in control sera.[19,20] Preliminary data have also shown significantly higher serum levels of zonulin in NCWS patients than in IBS patients and healthy control subjects. Although serum zonulin levels in NCWS did not differ from those found in CD, they tended to normalize more rapidly in the former than in the latter condition after GFD.[48] Another interesting finding comes from the study of mast cell density in the duodenal mucosa/submucosa. Our unpublished results indicate a higher mast cell density in NCWS in comparison with healthy control subjects and CD patients. This increased mast cell number in NCWS seems to be closely related with the presence of IBS-like symptoms, such as bloating, abdominal pain, and impaired bowel function. Moreover, the close vicinity of mast cells and nerve fibers observed in these patients may have a role in the generation of symptoms, such as abdominal pain, via a neuroimmune mechanism. No association has yet been identified between NCWS and specific genetic markers. The only certainty is that NCWS is not associated with HLA-DQ2 and/or HLA-DQ8, which have a high negative predictive value for CD. The frequencies of HLA-DQ2 and/or HLA-DQ8 are generally not found to be substantially different between NCWS and healthy individuals (see **Table 1**).[17,23,31,36,37,39] Nevertheless, genetic testing for these alleles is useful for patients who have already commenced a restricted diet without ruling out CD diagnosis. In these patients, negativity for DQ2 and DQ8 allows for the exclusion of CD.[5–8] Obviously, a gluten challenge remains mandatory for the diagnosis of patients who are positive for the DQ2/DQ8 genetic predisposition for CD (**Fig. 2**).

From a histopathologic standpoint, the intestinal mucosa in NCWS displays a normal villus/crypt ratio (>3:1), with a preserved villus architecture. An increase in

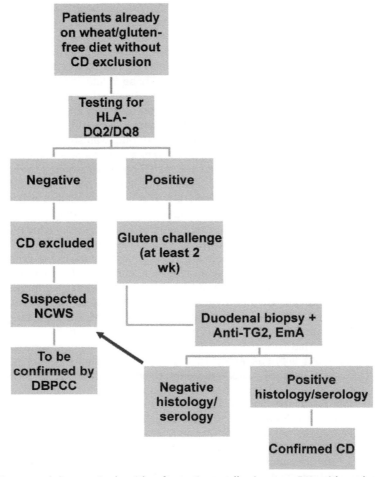

Fig. 2. Suggested diagnostic algorithm for patients adhering to a GFD without having previously ruled out celiac disease. Anti-TG2, anti–tissue transglutaminase; EmA, antiendomysial antibodies.

IELs, consistent with lesion type 1 according to the Marsh-Oberhüber classification, has been reported with a highly variable prevalence ranging from 26% to 96% of these patients (see **Table 1**).[17,24,32,44] In contrast to CD,[49] the IEL increase in NCWS is usually mild ranging from 25 to 40 lymphocytes in a high-power field.[31] Also, the distribution of lymphocytes might be helpful for differentiating NCWS from CD, because in the former these cells are located in the deeper part of the mucosa with a palisade pattern and in clusters in the villi, whereas in CD they are more closely confined to the epithelium with a diffuse distribution.[50]

Because of the current lack of established biomarkers, DBPCC is still regarded as the gold standard for confirming the diagnosis of NCWS.[5–8] However, this approach is not well accepted by patients who are already on a diet that excludes gluten-containing foods, while being time-consuming and difficult to implement. A review of 10 DBPCCs, including 1312 adults with IBS and/or suspected NCWS, revealed the lack of standardization.[51] In fact, the trials differed from one another for the selection of patients, the dosage of gluten or wheat, the duration of challenge (from 1 day to 6 weeks), and the composition of placebo (gluten-free products, xylose, whey protein, rice, or corn starch containing fermentable carbohydrates).[52] This systematic review of the literature suggested that only 16% of the patients evaluated by DBPCC for suspected NCWS experienced gluten-specific symptoms (triggered with gluten, but not with placebo ingestion).[51] The results emerging from the single studies confirmed a large variability in the rate of NCWS. Carroccio and colleagues[24] reported a prevalence of wheat sensitivity in 70 (26%) of 270 patients, whereas a further trial confirmed this diagnosis in 9 out of 59 (15%) patients, with three NCWS patients (5%) showing a particularly pronounced symptomatic response to gluten challenge.[52] More recently, NCWS was reported by means of DBPCC in 14% and 34% out of 98 and 35 patients, respectively.[53,54] Two trials carried out by the same investigative group produced somewhat different results with a first study (performed without crossover) confirming NCWS in 68% of cases,[55] and a second one (with crossover) finding it in only 8%.[56] Another recent study on a cohort of NCWS patients suggested that fructan oligosaccharides (a FODMAP) are the more likely culprits in the generation of intestinal symptoms (specifically bloating) when compared with gluten proteins.[57] The fructan used in the study originated from chicory roots, so it remains to be seen whether the actual fructo-oligosaccharide in wheat have the same effect. The study's findings also suggested that neither gluten proteins nor FODMAPs are by themselves significant triggers of the abdominal pain or extraintestinal symptoms associated with NCWS. Indeed, fructans can plausibly contribute to certain IBS-like symptoms, such as bloating, but they are less likely to be directly linked to immune activation or the extraintestinal symptoms associated with NCWS.[58] Furthermore, a role for the FODMAP (eg, fructans) component of wheat as the sole trigger for symptoms is somewhat doubtful, because many patients with NCWS report resolution of symptoms after the withdrawal of wheat and related cereals, while continuing to ingest vegetables and fruits with high FODMAP content in their diets.[59] On the whole, it is conceivable that more than one culprit may be involved in symptoms of NCWS (as they are currently defined), including gluten, other wheat proteins, and FODMAPs.[60–62] Five out of six DBPCC trials enrolling a total of 558 patients have confirmed the existence of NCWS, while suggesting that the frequency of the condition may be somewhat overestimated (**Table 2**) because of associated placebo effect. A further element supporting the existence of such wheat sensitivity comes from a study using confocal laser endomicroscopy.[63] The administration of wheat to the duodenal mucosa through the endoscopic route was found to induce small intestinal changes characterized by

Table 2
Study design and results of DBPCC for NCWS diagnosis

Reference	Study Design	Inclusion Criteria	Mode of Administration of Gluten/Wheat	Placebo	Duration of the Trial	Number of Patients Completing DBPCC	Number of Patients Having Symptoms Triggered with Gluten/Wheat but Not with Placebo
Biesiekierski et al,[56] 2013 Australia	Crossover randomized DBPCC	Self-reported NCWS patients	Food with high (16 g/d) or low content (2 g/d) of carbohydrate-depleted wheat protein	Gluten-free food with whey protein (16 g/d)	2-wk run-in period with a low-FODMAPs diet/ 1 wk with high- or low-gluten diet or placebo/2-wk wash-out before crossover for 1 wk	37	3 (8%)
Carroccio et al,[24] 2012, Italy	Crossover, randomized DBPCC	IBS and self-reported NCWS patients	Wheat flour–containing capsules (13 g/d)	Xylose-containing capsules	2 wk with one type of capsules/1-wk washout/2 wk with the other type of capsules	270	70 (26%)
Zanini et al,[54] 2015, Italy	Crossover randomized DBPCC	Self-reported NCWS patients	Gluten-containing flour	Gluten-free flour	10 d with one type of flour/2-wk wash-out/2 wk with the other flour	35	12 (34%)

Di Sabatino et al,[52] 2015, Italy	Crossover randomized DBPCC	Self-reported NCWS patients	Gluten-containing capsules (4.375 g/d)	Rice starch–containing capsules	1 wk with one type of capsules/1 wk wash-out/1 wk with the other type of capsules	9 (15%)[a]
Elli et al,[53] 2016, Italy	Crossover randomized DBPCC	Patients with functional symptoms, including IBS and functional dyspepsia	Gluten-containing capsules (5.6 g/d)	Rice starch–containing capsules	1 wk with one type of capsules/1 wk wash-out/1 wk with the other type of capsules	14 (14%)
Skodje et al,[57] 2018, Norway	Crossover randomized DBPCC	Self-reported NCWS patients	Gluten (5.7 g/d), fructans (2.1 g/d) concealed in muesli bars	Not reported	1 wk with one type of bars (once daily) with gluten or fructans or placebo, followed by 1-wk washout	0[b]
Overall results						108 (19.3%)

Results of DBPCC in patients with suspected NCWS: study design and modality of gluten/wheat administration, duration of the trial, number of patients completing the trial, and percentage of patients with confirmed NCWS (complaining of symptoms triggered with wheat/gluten and not with placebo).

[a] Of these patients, 3 of 59 (5%) showed a particularly pronounced symptomatic response to gluten.

[b] Fructans (not gluten) induced the highest symptom scores for bloating compared with placebo, but not for other NCWS-related symptoms.

increased IEL number, epithelial leaks/gaps, and widened intervillus spaces in more than one-third of the patients tested.

MANAGEMENT OF NONCELIAC WHEAT SENSITIVITY

The first recommendation for patients complaining of symptoms after the ingestion of gluten-containing food is to start the diagnostic work-up for CD and wheat allergy before any dietary restriction.[5–8] As recommended in the Fourth Consensus Conference on NCWS,[8] only after having ruled out both CD and wheat allergy should these patients be studied by an open trial of wheat/rye/barley-free diet for 6 weeks. Those who respond to the diet with the reduction of at least 30% in three symptoms based on the modified version of the GSRS[7] can be regarded as affected by suspected NCWS and should be kept on a diet that excludes wheat, rye, and barley, while awaiting further confirmation by a standardized DBPCC. The diagnosis of NCWS is excluded in those patients who do not improve after the wheat withdrawal. The DBPCC standardization is still far from being accomplished. In the third Consensus Conference on NCWS, an attempt to standardize a gluten-related challenge was undertaken.[7] It was recommended to test the patients with a gluten amount of 8 g/day, using a muesli bar as vehicle. Moreover, it was established that the ATI content should not be higher than 0.3 g/day and that the gluten vehicle should be without fructans. Another relevant input was that the gluten and placebo preparations should be indistinguishable in look and taste. A 1-week gluten challenge was recommended followed by a 1-week GFD and crossover to the second 1-week challenge. The diagnosis of NCWS could be confirmed when at least a variation of 30% between the gluten and placebo challenge is detected. By using the Salerno criteria, a recent DBPCC confirmed the existence of true NCWS in 11 out of 36 children (39.2%).[64]

FUTURE DIRECTIONS

Despite the clinical evidence for its existence and strong recent evidence for a biologic basis, NCWS is still a "work-in-progress" disorder with many unanswered questions.[65] Based on the clinical evidence available, gluten is thought to be relevant, but not the only culprit of this syndrome. Other components of wheat, such as ATIs and wheat germ agglutinins, and fructans (ie, FODMAPs), may have a role in symptom generation.[61–63] For this reason, the term NCWS seems to be preferable to nonceliac gluten sensitivity,[59] with the understanding that "wheat" also represents the closely related rye and barley, in the same way that the term "gluten" is now used to refer to the prolamin proteins of not only wheat, but also rye and barley. Because it is feasible to separate the different fractions of wheat and other related cereals, a DBPCC trial with five arms including pure preparations of gluten, ATIs, and fructans, and a complete wheat composition and placebo, could be a major step toward deciphering the impact of the different fractions of wheat in the clinical picture of NCWS. One of the most important challenges for the scientific community is the identification of established biomarkers for confirming the diagnosis without the need for DBPCC as already achieved for CD. Serum intestinal cell damage and immune activation markers have already given promising results, showing that the combination of several markers (AGA, LPS binding protein, sCD14, antibodies to LPS and flagellin, and FABP2) allows for the differentiation of NCWS from CD and control subjects with some outliers.[15] Other studies dealing with further characterization and validation of these biomarkers and possibly others, including those directly related to the small intestinal mucosa of NCWS patients, can improve the diagnostic work-up of this condition. Other potentially useful markers might be represented by the increased duodenal mast cell density interacting with nerve fibers as a potential trigger for symptom generation. The identification of biomarkers will also allow for clarification of the prevalence of NCWS, which is currently based on estimates using various assumptions.[66] Another unanswered question is whether NCWS is a disorder with possible recovery like wheat allergy or a primarily permanent condition like CD. Although still debatable, a recent study suggests that NCWS may be a chronic disorder.[67] Of 200 patients with NCWS confirmed by DBPCC and followed up for 8 years, 148 were still on the restricted diet, whereas 52 came back to a gluten-containing diet. Ninety-eight percent of those still on a restricted diet remained symptom-free compared with only 58% of those on a gluten-containing diet, suggesting that the reintroduction of gluten-containing foods was associated with a significantly higher recurrence of symptoms. **Table 3** summarizes the comparison among NCWS, CD, and IBS.

Table 3
Comparison for various features in IBS, NCWS, and CD

	IBS	NCWS	CD
Epidemiology	10%–20%	Unknown (possible range, 0.6%–6%)	1%
Duration	Chronic	Unknown	Chronic
Pathogenesis	Multifactorial (innate immunity involved)	Innate immunity	Innate/adaptive immunity
Onset age	40–50 y	30–40 y	Any age
Gender	Female/male 2:1	Female/male 5:1	Female/male 2:1
Familiarity for gluten-related disorders	Variable	Present	Present
Symptoms	Gastrointestinal	Gastrointestinal/ extraintestinal	Gastrointestinal/ extraintestinal
Biomarkers	None	None (AGA?)	Anti-tTG and EmA
HLA	None	None	HLA-DQ2 and HLA-DQ8 restricted
Duodenal histology	Normal mucosa	Normal mucosa/mild lesions	Villus atrophy
Autoimmune disorders	Low prevalence	High prevalence	High prevalence
Reduced bone mineral density		Up to 50%	Up to 70%
Food intolerance	Lactose intolerance	Lactose/fructose intolerance	Lactose/fructose intolerance
Outcome (complications)	No complications	No complications	Refractory disease, lymphoma, small bowel adenocarcinoma, ulcerative jejunoileitis
DBPCC	Unnecessary for diagnosis	Recommended for diagnosis	Unnecessary for diagnosis

Comparison of epidemiologic, pathogenic, clinical, diagnostic, and outcome features of IBS, NCWS, and CD.
Abbreviations: Anti-tTG, antibodies to tissue transglutaminase; EmA, antiendomysial antibodies.

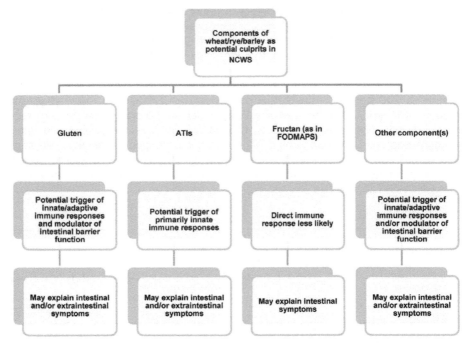

Fig. 3. Different components of wheat, such as gluten, fructans (as part of FODMAPs), ATIs, and other molecules, may act as triggers of NCWS, including immune system modulation, intestinal barrier disruption, and symptom generation.

SUMMARY

Interest in NCWS within the scientific community is reflected by the increasing number of original papers, reviews, and trials published on this topic in the past 10 years. The initial skepticism surrounding this disorder has gradually given way to a progressing awareness of the existence of NCWS. This diagnosis has been confirmed by DBPCC trials in varying proportions of patients with self-reported NCWS.[51] The exact triggers among the various components of wheat and related cereals for the associated symptoms remains unclear, but gluten, ATIs, and fructan, and other components, may play a role.[60–62] FODMAPs have been reported to contribute to certain intestinal symptoms in some patients with NCWS, but other components of wheat and related cereals, such as specific proteins, are believed to trigger substantial immune activation and/or intestinal barrier dysfunction that would explain gastrointestinal and extraintestinal manifestations **(Fig. 3)**.[58] The identification and confirmation of established biomarkers is eagerly awaited because their availability will allow for the diagnosis of this condition without the need for time-consuming food challenge, which is not well-accepted by patients. Promising results have been achieved by the analysis of markers of intestinal cell damage and systemic immune activation. Further evaluation of the mechanisms involved in the generation of these markers is likely to add significantly to the understanding of NCWS and the identification of associated diagnostic markers.

REFERENCES

1. Leonard MM, Sapone A, Catassi C, et al. Celiac disease and nonceliac gluten sensitivity: a review. JAMA 2017;318:647–56.

2. Lebwohl B, Sanders DS, Green PHR. Coeliac disease. Lancet 2018;391:70–81.
3. Volta U, De Giorgio R. New understanding of gluten sensitivity. Nat Rev Gastroenterol Hepatol 2012;9:295–9.
4. Lebwohl B, Ludvigsson JF, Green PH. Celiac disease and non-celiac gluten sensitivity. BMJ 2015;351: h4347.
5. Sapone A, Bai JC, Ciacci C, et al. Spectrum of gluten-related disorders: consensus on new nomenclature and classification. BMC Med 2012;10:13.
6. Catassi C, Bai JC, Bonaz B, et al. Non-celiac gluten sensitivity: the new frontier of gluten related disorders. Nutrients 2013;5:3839–53.
7. Catassi C, Elli L, Bonaz B, et al. Diagnosis of non-celiac gluten sensitivity (NCGS): the Salerno Experts' Criteria. Nutrients 2015;7:4966–77.
8. Catassi C, Alaedini A, Bojarski C, et al. The overlapping area of non-celiac gluten sensitivity (NCGS) and wheat-sensitive irritable bowel syndrome (IBS): an update. Nutrients 2017;9(11) [pii:E1268].
9. Junker Y, Zeissig S, Kim SJ, et al. Wheat amylase trypsin inhibitors drive intestinal inflammation via activation of toll-like receptor 4. J Exp Med 2012;209:2395–408.
10. De Giorgio R, Volta U, Gibson PR. Sensitivity to wheat, gluten and FODMAPs in IBS: facts or fiction? Gut 2016;65:169–78.
11. Di Sabatino A, Corazza GR. Nonceliac gluten sensitivity: sense or sensibility? Ann Intern Med 2012;156:309–11.
12. Suarez FL, Savaiano DA, Levitt MD. A comparison of symptoms after the consumption of milk or lactose-hydrolyzed milk by people with self-reported severe lactose intolerance. N Engl J Med 1995;333:1–4.
13. Molina-Infante J, Santolaria S, Sanders DS, et al. Systematic review: non-coeliac gluten sensitivity. Aliment Pharmacol Ther 2015;41:807–20.
14. Volta U, Caio G, Karunaratne TB, et al. Non-coeliac gluten/wheat sensitivity: advances in knowledge and relevant questions. Expert Rev Gastroenterol Hepatol 2017;11:9–18.
15. Uhde M, Ajamian M, Caio G, et al. Intestinal cell damage and systemic immune activation in individuals reporting sensitivity to wheat in the absence of coeliac disease. Gut 2016;65:1930–7.
16. Fasano A, Sapone A, Zevallos V, et al. Non-celiac gluten sensitivity. Gastroenterology 2015;149:1195–204.
17. Sapone A, Lammers KM, Casolaro V, et al. Divergence of gut permeability and mucosal immune gene expression in two gluten associated conditions: celiac disease and gluten sensitivity. BMC Med 2011;9:23.
18. Vazquez-Roque MI, Camilleri M, Smyrk T, et al. A controlled trial of gluten-free diet in patients with irritable bowel syndrome-diarrhea: effects on bowel frequency and intestinal function. Gastroenterology 2013;144:903–11.
19. Valerii MC, Ricci C, Spisni E, et al. Responses of peripheral blood mononucleated cells from non-celiac gluten sensitive patients to various cereal sources. Food Chem 2015;176:167–74.
20. Alvisi P, De Fazio L, Valerii MC, et al. Responses of blood mononucleated cells and clinical outcome of non-celiac gluten sensitive pediatric patients to various cereal sources: a pilot study. Int J Food Sci Nutr 2017;68:1005–12.
21. Di Liberto D, Mansueto P, D'Alcamo A, et al. Predominance of type 1 innate lymphoid cells in the rectal mucosa of patients with non-celiac wheat sensitivity: reversal after a wheat-free diet. Clin Transl Gastroenterol 2016;7:e178.
22. Brottveit M, Beitnes AC, Tollefsen S, et al. Mucosal cytokine response after short-term gluten challenge in celiac disease and non-celiac gluten sensitivity. Am J Gastroenterol 2013;108:842–50.

23. Volta U, Tovoli F, Cicola R, et al. Serological tests in gluten sensitivity (nonceliac gluten intolerance). J Clin Gastroenterol 2012;46:680–5.
24. Carroccio A, Mansueto P, Iacono G, et al. Non-celiac wheat sensitivity diagnosed by double-blind placebo-controlled challenge: exploring a new clinical entity. Am J Gastroenterol 2012;107:1898–906.
25. Wu RL, Vazquez-Roque MI, Carlson P, et al. Gluten-induced symptoms in diarrhea-predominant irritable bowel syndrome are associated with increased myosin light chain kinase activity and claudin-15 expression. Lab Invest 2017; 97:14–23.
26. Dieterich W, Schuppan D, Schink M, et al. Influence of low FODMAP and gluten-free diets on disease activity and intestinal microbiota in patients with non-celiac gluten sensitivity. Clin Nutr 2018. [Epub ahead of print].
27. Pozo-Rubio T, Olivares M, Nova E, et al. Immune development and intestinal microbiota in celiac disease. Clin Dev Immunol 2012;2012:654143.
28. Saulnier DM, Riehle K, Mistretta TA, et al. Gastrointestinal microbiome signatures of pediatric patients with irritable bowel syndrome. Gastroenterology 2011 Nov; 14:1782–91.
29. Manichanh C, Borruel N, Casellas F, et al. The gut microbiota in IBD. Nat Rev Gastroenterol Hepatol 2012;9:599–608.
30. DiGiacomo DV, Tennyson CA, Green PH, et al. Prevalence of gluten-free diet adherence among individuals without celiac disease in the USA: results from the Continuous National Health and Nutrition Examination Survey 2009-2010. Scand J Gastroenterol 2013;48:921–5.
31. Volta U, Bardella MT, Calabrò A, et al. An Italian prospective multicenter survey on patients suspected of having non-celiac gluten sensitivity. BMC Med 2014; 12:85.
32. Hadjivassiliou M, Rao DG, Grünewald RA, et al. Neurological dysfunction in coeliac disease and non-coeliac gluten sensitivity. Am J Gastroenterol 2016; 111:561–7.
33. Rodrigo L, Blanco I, Bobes J, et al. Effect of one year of a gluten-free diet on the clinical evolution of irritable bowel syndrome plus fibromyalgia in patients with associated lymphocytic enteritis: a case-control study. Arthritis Res Ther 2014; 16:421.
34. Bonciolini V, Bianchi B, Del Bianco E, et al. Cutaneous manifestations of non-coeliac gluten sensitivity: clinical, histological and immunopathological features. Nutrients 2015;7:7798–805.
35. Carroccio A, Soresi M, D'Alcamo A, et al. Risk of low bone mineral density and low body mass index in patients with non-celiac wheat-sensitivity: a prospective observation study. BMC Med 2014;12:230.
36. Aziz I, Lewis NR, Hadjivassiliou M, et al. A UK study assessing the population prevalence of self-reported gluten sensitivity and referral characteristics to secondary care. Eur J Gastroenterol Hepatol 2014;26:33–9.
37. Kabbani TA, Vanga RR, Leffler DA, et al. Celiac disease or non-celiac gluten sensitivity? An approach to clinical differential diagnosis. Am J Gastroenterol 2014;109:741–6.
38. Carroccio A, Brusca I, Mansueto P, et al. A comparison between two different in vitro basophil activation tests for gluten- and cow's milk protein sensitivity in irritable bowel syndrome (IBS)-like patients. Clin Chem Lab Med 2013;51:1257–63.
39. Carroccio A, D'Alcamo A, Cavataio F, et al. High proportions of people with non-celiac wheat sensitivity have autoimmune disease or antinuclear antibodies. Gastroenterology 2015;149:596–603.

40. Volta U, Caio G, De Giorgio R. Is autoimmunity more predominant in nonceliac wheat sensitivity than celiac disease? Gastroenterology 2016;150:282.

41. Volta U, Villanacci V. Celiac disease: diagnostic criteria in progress. Cell Mol Immunol 2011;8:96–102.

42. Inomata N. Wheat allergy. Curr Opin Allergy Clin Immunol 2009;9:238–43.

43. Francavilla R, Cristofori F, Castellaneta S, et al. Clinical, serologic, and histologic features of gluten sensitivity in children. J Pediatr 2014;164:463–7.

44. Volta U, Granito A, Parisi C, et al. Deamidated gliadin peptide antibodies as a routine test for celiac disease: a prospective analysis. J Clin Gastroenterol 2010;44:186–90.

45. Caio G, Volta U, Tovoli F, et al. Effect of gluten free diet on immune response to gliadin in patients with non-celiac gluten sensitivity. BMC Gastroenterol 2014; 14:26.

46. Uhde M, Caio G, De Giorgio R, et al. Serologic markers of systemic immune activation and intestinal cell damage in non-celiac wheat sensitivity. Gastroenterology 2017;152(S1):S37.

47. Uhde M, Indart AC, Yu XB, et al. Markers of non-coeliac wheat sensitivity in patients with myalgic encephalomyelitis/chronic fatigue syndrome. Gut 2018. [Epub ahead of print].

48. Barbaro MR, Cremon C, Caio G, et al. Increased zonulin serum levels and correlation with symptoms in non-celiac gluten sensitivity and irritable bowel syndrome with diarrhea. United European J Gastroenterol 2014;2(suppl. 1):A555.

49. Rostami K, Marsh MN, Johnson MW, et al. ROC-king onwards: intraepithelial lymphocyte counts, distribution & role in coeliac disease mucosal interpretation. Gut 2017;66:2080–6.

50. Zanini B, Villanacci V, Marullo M, et al. Duodenal histological features in suspected non-celiac gluten sensitivity: new into a still undefined condition. Virchows Arch 2018;473(2):229–34.

51. Molina-Infante J, Carroccio A. Suspected nonceliac gluten sensitivity confirmed in few patients after gluten challenge in double-blind, placebo-controlled trials. Clin Gastroenterol Hepatol 2017;15:339–48.

52. Di Sabatino A, Volta U, Salvatore C, et al. Small amounts of gluten in subjects with suspected nonceliac gluten sensitivity: a randomized, double-blind, placebo-controlled, cross-over trial. Clin Gastroenterol Hepatol 2015;13:1604–12.

53. Elli L, Tomba C, Bianchi F, et al. Evidence for the presence of non-coeliac gluten sensitivity in patients with functional gastrointestinal symptoms: results form a multicenter randomized double-blind placebo-controlled gluten challenge. Nutrients 2016;8:84.

54. Zanini B, Baschè R, Ferraresi A, et al. Randomised clinical study: gluten challenge induces symptom recurrence in only a minority of patients who meet clinical criteria for non-coeliac gluten sensitivity. Aliment Pharmacol Ther 2015;42: 968–76.

55. Biesiekierski JR, Newnham ED, Irving PM, et al. Gluten causes gastrointestinal symptoms in subjects without celiac disease: a double-blind randomized placebo-controlled trial. Am J Gastroenterol 2011;106:508–14.

56. Biesiekierski JR, Peters SL, Newnham ED, et al. No effects of gluten in patients with self-reported non-celiac gluten sensitivity after dietary reduction of fermentable, poorly absorbed, short-chain carbohydrates. Gastroenterology 2013;145: 320–8.

57. Skodje GI, Sarna VK, Minelle IH, et al. Fructan, rather than gluten, induces symptoms in patients with self-reported non-celiac gluten sensitivity. Gastroenterology 2018;154:529–39.
58. Verbeke K. Nonceliac gluten sensitivity: what is the culprit? Gastroenterology 2018;154:471–3.
59. Prichard R, Rossi M, Muir J, et al. Fermentable oligosaccharide, disaccharide, monosaccharide and polyol content of foods commonly consumed by ethnic minority groups in the United Kingdom. Int J Food Sci Nutr 2016;67:383–90.
60. Schuppan D, Pickert G, Ashfaq-Khan M, et al. Non-celiac wheat sensitivity: differential diagnosis, triggers and implications. Best Pract Res Clin Gastroenterol 2015;29:469–76.
61. de Punder K, Pruimboom L. The dietary intake of wheat and other cereal grains and their role in inflammation. Nutrients 2013;5:771–87.
62. Halmos EP, Power VA, Shepherd SJ, et al. A diet low in FODMAPs reduces symptoms of irritable bowel syndrome. Gastroenterology 2014;146:67–75.
63. Fritscher-Ravens A, Schuppan D, Ellrichmann M, et al. Confocal endomicroscopy shows food-associated changes in the intestinal mucosa of patients with irritable bowel syndrome. Gastroenterology 2014;147:1012–20.
64. Francavilla R, Cristofori F, Verzillo L, et al. Randomized double-blind placebo-controlled crossover trial for the diagnosis of non-celiac gluten sensitivity in children. Am J Gastroenterol 2018;113(3):421–30.
65. Volta U, Caio G, De Giorgio R, et al. Non-celiac gluten sensitivity: a work-in-progress entity in the spectrum of wheat-related disorders. Best Pract Res Clin Gastroenterol 2015;29:477–91.
66. Vasagar B, Cox J, Herion JT, et al. World epidemiology of non-celiac gluten sensitivity. Minerva Gastroenterol Dietol 2017;63:5–15.
67. Carroccio A, D'Alcamo A, Iacono G, et al. Persistence of nonceliac wheat sensitivity, based on long-term follow-up. Gastroenterology 2017;153:56–8.

Moving?

Make sure your subscription moves with you!

To notify us of your new address, find your **Clinics Account Number** (located on your mailing label above your name), and contact customer service at:

Email: journalscustomerservice-usa@elsevier.com

800-654-2452 (subscribers in the U.S. & Canada)
314-447-8871 (subscribers outside of the U.S. & Canada)

Fax number: 314-447-8029

Elsevier Health Sciences Division
Subscription Customer Service
3251 Riverport Lane
Maryland Heights, MO 63043

*To ensure uninterrupted delivery of your subscription, please notify us at least 4 weeks in advance of move.

Printed and bound by CPI Group (UK) Ltd, Croydon, CR0 4YY

03/10/2024

01040405-0014